EATING HEALTHY GOD'S WAY

The Pathway to a Life Free of Food Borne Disease

A basic guide to applying the principles of

Nutrition and diet as set forth in the Holy Bible

Author Oliver Smith

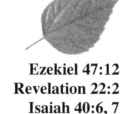

Ezekiel 47:12
Revelation 22:2
Isaiah 40:6, 7

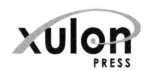

Copyright © 2011 by Oliver Smith

Eating Healthy God's Way
The Pathway to a Life Free of Food Borne Disease
by Oliver Smith

Printed in the United States of America

ISBN 9781613799253

All rights reserved solely by the author. The author guarantees all contents are original and do not infringe upon the legal rights of any other person or work. No part of this book may be reproduced in any form without the permission of the author. The views expressed in this book are not necessarily those of the publisher.

Unless otherwise indicated, all scripture quotations are taken from the King James Version of the Holy Bible.

Scripture quotations identified as New Spirit Filled Life Bible are taken from the New Spirit Filled Life Bible.

www.xulonpress.com

TABLE OF CONTENTS

Disclaimer	ix
Dedication, Acknowledgments, Preface & Introduction	xi-xvii
The Vision	19
The Apple	20
Violation of God's Principles / John 8:32	21
Spring Water	22
Nutritional Negatives / Irritants / Foods to Avoid	23
Seeded Grapes	25
Dr. Dwight Lundell, Cholesterol & Heart Disease	26
What is inflammation?	30
Vegetable Photos	31
Fruit Photo	32
Eight GMO Foods should never eat	33
Berry Photo	34
Seeded Watermelon Photo	35
The Watermelon You Should Never, Ever Eat	36
Watermelon, Seeded Photo	40
Wild Natural Garlic	41
Photo of Vegetables	42
CDC, Center for Disease Control	43
Wild Locust	44
Black Pepper & Cancer	45
The US Dept. Of Agriculture / meat safety cooking chart	46
Grass Fed Cattle Photo	47
100% Grass Fed Natural Beef / Nutritional Analysis / Slanker's Meats	48
Grass Fed & Non Grass Fed Cattle	50
Butter From Grass Fed Cattle	51
Free Range Chickens & Eggs, God's Basket	52-54
100% Grass Fed Lamb	55
Grass Fed Goats	58
Goats Milk & Cheese	59
White Tail Deer	60
Wild Turkeys, Natural Feed	61

Wild Partridge	62
Wild Caught Fish by Bear	63
Vegetable & Fruit Photo	64
All Natural Almond Trees & Almonds	65
All Natural Cucumbers	67
Chain of Life, Enzymes	68
Wild Honey & Bee	69
Photo of All Natural Stevia Plant	70
What are the Benefits of Stevia	71
Stevia in the Raw, Sweetness Substitution Chart	74
Sugars & Substitutes with their Glycemic Index Chart	75
Green Leafy Vegetable Photo	78
Foods That Promote Cleansing	79
Natural Organic Bean Photo	81
The Origin of the Word Vegetables	82
Photo of Vegetable Field	83
Did You Know? Leaf Vegetables	84
Foods Authorized by the Holy Scriptures, KJV	85
About Natural Weight Control, Did You Know?	88
Vegetable Photo	89
US Senate Doc. No. 264 • • • **Top Secret** • • •	**90**
Introduction to a Collection of Healthy Recipes	100

BREAKFAST

Ezekiel Blueberry Pancakes	101
French Toast Ezekiel Bread	102
Grapefruit & Eggs	103
Heaven's Breakfast	104
Eggs Sunnyside Up with Ezekiel Toast	105
Divine Breakfast	106
Breakfast from God's Garden	107

ENTREES

CCC Salmon Salad	108
Broiled Beef Steak	109
Garlic Chicken	110
Broiled Salmon Fillets	111
Sea Bass Broiled With Salad	112
Broiled Lamb Chops	113
Daniel's Salad	114
Cheese Burger on Ezekiel Bun	115
Hamburger on Ezekiel Bun	116
Summary	117

The Centerpoint of Nutrition, 90 Essential Nutrients 119
Recommended Reading 120

GOD's GROCERY STORE 121
Where to find natural foods.. 122
God's Natural Spring Waters 123

Closing Prayer... 126

Albert Einstein: God, Religion & Theology 127

None of the foods, food components, substances or products mentioned in this book in and of themselves cure or heal anything. And there is no statement made herein to say otherwise, and none are implied or intended. Such supplemental foods, supplements, nutriceuticals, botanicals (herbs) and phytonutrients simply function as foods do, which is to nourish the body – and, therefore, - they simply aid the body to function and operate normally, and facilitate the body's own inherent ability to fix itself.

All products listed in this book are categorized as foods, nutritional supplements, botanicals (herbs), and / or functional foods and nutriceuticals within the guidelines and standards set by the U.S. Food & Drug Administration FDA, and as also regulated by the U.S. Federal Trade Commission FTC with regard to what can be said about them in accordance with current law. All the products listed herein, furthermore, are generally regarded as inherently non-toxic by current government, industry, and/or historical standards.

DEDICATION

"This book is dedicated to Jesus Christ, the son of God. God who is our provider, and who is our all bountiful supplier, he is also the Lord our healer. The Lord our God has supplied us, his children with the Holy Bible which tells us which foods are clean and edible and which foods are unclean and we are forbidden to eat. The principles and instructions set forth in the Holy Bible would certainly keep us free of food borne diseases if obeyed. I am thankful to God for the principles and instructions set forth in the Holy Bible that allows us to experience abundant health and life. I shall spend the rest of my time on earth sharing that which I have learned that will bring the sort of health that God planned for man, when God created man in his image and his likeness. OH! WHAT A MIGHTY GOD WE SERVE!"

Let all things be done decently and in order. 1 Corinthians 14:40

Take fast hold of instruction; let her not go: keep her; for she is thy life. Proverbs 4:13

All scripture is given by inspiration of God, and is profitable for doctrine, for reproof, for correction, for instruction in righteousness. 2 Timothy 3:16

Acknowledgments

The first grateful acknowledgment and praise is to God. Without God we would not have the Holy Bible. Without the Holy Bible, we would not have the list of foods authorized by God. Without the Holy Bible we would not know that the seventh year shall be a Sabbath of rest unto the land and laborers as well. Without the Holy Bible we would not know God's principles and instructions that would lead us to a life free of food borne disease. Glory to God.

Many people have helped with this project. This book has been produced in a short amount of time, though it is an accumulation of years of research. A special acknowledgment must go out to certain people who have put in long strenuous hours to have this book become fruition.

I gratefully acknowledge Pastor Phillip G. Goudeaux. Pastor Goudeaux is an example of a true leader of men directed by the word of God. Pastor Goudeaux has long believed that the food borne diseases that claim the lives of too many Christians prematurely can only occur by a violation of God's Principles and instructions. This book was put together with the intent of providing a list of foods as set forth by God from the Holy Scriptures. The belief is that God would not provide food that would be harmful to his people. The Holy Bible gave us the dots, now we must connect the dots in order to live a life free of food borne disease. We simply needed to fine the dots. Pastor Goudeaux provided the inspiration for the research and writing. Peter McAllister, Pastor's executive assistant provided the whip, thanks Peter. Thank God for vision Pastor Goudeaux's vision.

I gratefully acknowledge Dr. Joel Wallach for providing the guidelines set forth by his many years of experience in forensic science and wholistic health and his love for God. Thank you Dr. Wallach.

I gratefully acknowledge Minister Vivian Hodge, Certified Wholistic Health Consultant, (Iridology, Nutrition, Herbology.) Minister Hodge is a wealth of knowledge regarding the Holy Scriptures and health. Thanks Vivian for taking my calls and directing my efforts.

I gratefully acknowledge Pamela Johnson of pjwebdesignz (http://www.pjzwebdesignz.com.) Pamela's computer consulting skills were irreplaceable. Thank Pam.

I gratefully acknowledge Dr. Michael Monroe, minister, teacher, friend and great spiritual leader. May God bless you Dr. Monroe.

I gratefully acknowledge Brenda Boudreaux, attorney, journalist and friend for her assistance with the cover of this book. Thanks Brenda.

A special thanks to my daughter Olivia Smith, who believes her Dad, can do anything. Thanks to my son Joey who is an EMT in the US Army. Thank you for your service my son. I love you two.

Preface

The principle behind the foods that God provides his people promotes health and healing.

> **…leaf there of for Medicine;**
> - **Ezekiel 47:12** and by the river upon the bank thereof, shall grow all tree for meat, and the fruit therefore shall be for meat, and the leaf thereof for medicine.
>
> **…leaves…healing of the nations;**
> - **Revelation 22:2** …and the leaves of the tree were for the healing of the nations.
>
> **…make thee bread;**
> - **Ezekiel 4:9** Take thou also unto thee wheat, and barley, and beans, and lentils, and millet, and fitches, and put them in one vessel, and make thee bread thereof, according to the number of the days that thou shalt lie upon thy side, three hundred and ninety days shalt thou eat thereof.
>
> **…all flesh is grass,…**
> - **Isaiah 40:6** …All flesh is grass, and all the goodliness thereof is as the flower of the field:
>
> - **Isaiah 40:7** the grass withereth, the flower fadeth: because the spirit of the Lord bloweth upon it: surely the people is grass.

Introduction

This is a book by a legal researcher / investigator / paralegal / nutritionist / naturalist and consultant, whose background, training and experience as a child of God qualify him uniquely to write for the public as well as the Christian Community regarding food provided for man by God.

This is also a book that is grossly overdue and vital to the well being of all God's people in America and around the world who are suffering from the affect of the food borne diseases. Question, would God our creator provide food with the intent to destroy the human body? Of course not, then why and how are so many people suffering and dying from food borne diseases?

As a trained and experienced researcher I believe the Holy Bible provides the answers and science provides evidences of truth regarding the answers to these two questions.

- **1 Corinthians 6:19** …know ye not that your body is the temple of the Holy Ghost which is in you, which ye have of God, and ye are not your own?

    You do not belong to you. Your body is the temple of the Holy Ghost. You are a steward of God's property. As a steward of God's property, we have a divine responsibility to keep our bodies well and free of any food borne disease.

- **1 Corinthians 6:20** For ye are bought with a price: therefore glorify God in your body, and in your Spirit, which are God's.

…GOD IN YOUR BODY, AND IN YOUR SPIRIT, WHICH ARE GOD'S.

- **Proverbs 3:5** Trust in the Lord with all thine heart: and lean not unto thine own understanding.

…LEAN NOT UNTO THINE OWN UNDERSTANDING.

- **Proverbs 3:6** In all thy ways acknowledge him, and he shall direct thy paths.

> - **Proverbs 3:7** Be not wise in thine own eyes: fear the Lord, and depart from evil.
>
> **BE NOT WISE IN THINE OWN EYES:...**
>
> - **Romans 13:14** But put on the Lord Jesus Christ, and make not provision for the flesh, to fulfill the lusts thereof.
>
> **...AND MAKE NOT PROVISION FOR THE FLESH...**
>
> - **Number 11:33** And while the flesh was yet between their teeth, ere it was chewed, the wrath of the Lord was kindled against the people, and the Lord smote the people with a very great plague.
>
> - **Number 11:34** And he called the name of that place Kib'-roth-hat-ta-a-vah: because there they buried the people that lusted.

Do not allow your taste buds to control your health by LUSTING after and eating foods that taste good, but lack nutritional value and becomes destructive to the human body once eaten.

Is it a sin to destroy God's property?

The Vision

God's plan and vision by Oliver Smith

God's vision is set forth in the Holy Bible. **Genesis 1:26** And God said, "Let us make man in our image, after our likeness:…" Dr Joel Wallach has been known to ask, "Do you have any images of God suffering alzheimer's disease, cancer, diabetes, constipation or hemorrhoids?" Of course not and neither would man or woman suffer these diseases, if they were to follow the laws, principles and instructions as set forth in The Holy Bible.

The further we live our lives from the laws, principles and instructions as set forth in our creator's owners manual designed and written for man, The Holy Bible! The further we are from the health and wellness that God had planned for us when he made us in his image and likeness.

The vision, that the members of the Christian Community in the United States of America and the world as well live a life free of food borne disease by honoring the word of God and his laws, principles and instructions.

Habakkuk 2:2 says, And the Lord answered me, and said write the vision, and make it plain upon tables, that he may run that readeth.

Proverbs 29:18 says, Where there is no vision, the people perish: but he that keepeth the law, happy is he.

"All scripture is given by inspiration of God, and is profitable for doctrine, for reproof, for correction, for instruction in righteousness."

2 Timothy 3:16

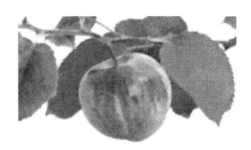

VIOLATION OF GOD'S PRINCIPLES

Leviticus 25:4 says, "But in the seventh year shall be a Sabbath of rest unto the land, a Sabbath for the Lord: thou shalt neither sow thy field, nor prune thy vineyard."

Leviticus 25:5 says, "That which growth of its own accord of thy harvest thou shalt not reap, neither gather the grapes of thy vine undressed: for it is a year of rest unto the land.

Violation of God's principles leads to destruction: we know that there is no, nor has there ever been, any rest unto the land in America.

See the article regarding the work of Dr. Charles Northen: Dr. Charles Northen builds health from the ground up.

TOP SECRET

Must read; Modern Miracle Men, Senate Document 264 hereto attached. (See table of contents)

John 8:32 And ye shall know the truth, and the truth shall make you free.

Make no mistake, be prepared to take action on what you learn here in this book, and you will experience the health that God planned for you.

Proverbs 9:6 says, "Forsake the foolish, and live; and go in the way of understanding."

Proverbs 9:9 says, "Give instruction to a wise man, and he will be yet wiser: teach a just man, and he will increase in learning."

"It is incumbent upon the children of God not to just talk about the truth, but to actually seek it, find it and to live it."

Anonymous child of God

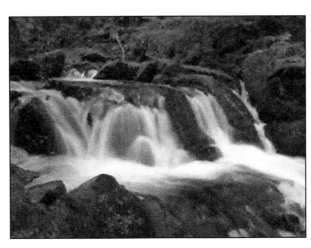

Isaiah 58:11 says, "And the Lord shall guide thee continually, and satisfy thy soul in drought, and make fat thy bones: and thou shall be like a watered garden, and like a spring of water, whose water fail not."

Proverbs 9:9, 10 says, "Give instruction to a wise man, and he will be yet wiser: teach a just man, and he will increase in learning. The fear of the Lord is the beginning of wisdom: and the knowledge of the holy is understanding."

Nutritional Negatives / Irritants
Foods to avoid

- All <u>carbonated drinks</u>, soda pop, in bottles as well as cans.
- **MARGARINE** is but 1 molecule from being plastic.
- Do not use artificial butter, imitation butter or butter substitutes.
- Processed **SUGARS**, artificial, imitation sugar & sugar substitutes.
- **GLUTENS**, all foods containing **WHEAT**, cakes, pies, cookies, breads and **CEREALS** including **OATMEAL**.
- Fried foods, **ALL HEATED OILS ARE KNOWN CARCINOGENIC**
- High fiber diets. Have been known to strip essential minerals from our bodies.
- Burnt and **OVER COOKED MEATS ARE KNOWN TO BE CARCINOGENIC**.
- All lunch meats containing sodium nitrate & sodium nitrite.
- All synthetic / artificial vitamins or nutrients.
- **GMO's, Genetically Modified Organisms (FOODS)**.
- Meat Glue, called Transglutaminase.

• • •Foods NOT Permitted to eat, per the Holy Bible• • •

- **Leviticus 3:17** It shall be a perpetual statute for your generations throughout all your dwellings, <u>that ye eat neither fat nor blood.</u>

- **Leviticus 6:23** For every meat offering for the priest shall be <u>wholly burnt: it shall not be eaten.</u>

- **Leviticus 7:23** Speak unto the children of Israel, saying, <u>Ye shall eat no manner of fat, of ox, or of sheep, or of goat.</u>

- **Leviticus 7:24-25-26** And the fat of the beast that dieth of itself, and the fat of that which is torn with beasts, may be used in any other use: <u>but ye shall in no wise eat of it. …eat no manner of blood</u>

- **Leviticus 11:1-6**, Now the Lord spoke to Moses and Aaron, saying to them, Speak unto the children of Israel, saying, These are the beasts which ye shall eat among all the beasts that are on the earth.

- **Leviticus 11:7** <u>And the swine</u>…, he is unclean to you.

> - **Leviticus 11:12** Whatsoever hath **no fins nor scales**... be an abomination unto you. (Recommended reading Leviticus 11:3-47)
>
> - **Deuteronomy 14:3-4-21** You shall not eat any detestable thing. ...the camel, and the hare, and the coney, the swine, nor touch their dead carcase. And whatsoever hath not fins and scales ye may not eat: ye shall not eat: the eagle, and the ossifrage, ospray, glede, and the kite, and the vulture after his kind, the raven after his kind, And theowl, and the night hawk, and the cuckow, and the hawk after his kind. The little owl, and the great owl, and the swan, pelican, and the gier eagle, the cormorant ye shall not eat. Ye shall not stork, and the heron after her kind, and lapwing, the bat ye shall eat.

God did NOT create any seedless grapes or water melons.

Consumer Report...

Hazardous non-stick coating

That's why many people opt for non-stick pots and pans even though they are not as durable as their aluminum or stainless steel counterparts. Within the past few years, several studies have started to illustrate the dangers of non-stick cookware. Ongoing research at the University of Toronto has influenced the U.S. Environmental Protection Agency (EPA) to outlaw the production of perfluorochemicals, the ingredients used to make Teflon, Stainmaster, and Gore-tex materials. Perfluorochemicals may give pots and pans that non-stick glide, but they are also carcinogenic. Fortunately, there are some new-generation non-stick options in the marketplace that are easy to use and to clean but don't contain the dangerous chemicals scientists are worried about.

Both the uncoated 8 Calphalon and 10 All-Clad delivered impressive cooking performance.

The Swiss Diamond Reinforced nonstick pans were the best performers overall but we didn't include them in the Select Ratings (available to subscribers) because of their $500 price tag. They do not contain PFOA, according to the manufacturer, which says the surface is a nanoparticle composite of diamond crystals.

The most expensive pots and pans we tested, the $830 All-Clad Copper Core 6000-7SS, scored only average in sturdiness and comfort of the handle. The bottom-ranked $300 Mercola Healthy Chef is made mostly of ceramic. In our tests, it burned food and two of its handles broke.

All natural seeded grapes

Leviticus 19:10 says, "And thou shalt not glean thy vineyard, neither shalt thou gather **every grape** of thy vineyard; thou shalt leave them for the poor and stranger: I am the Lord your God."

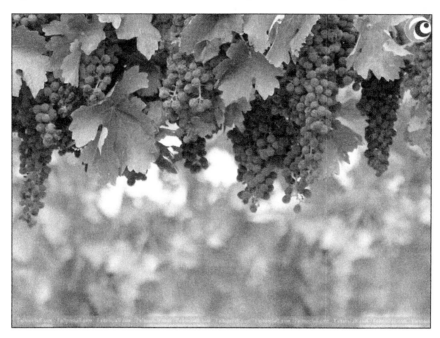

Cholesterol and Heart Disease

World Renown Heart Surgeon Speaks Out On What Really Causes Heart Disease

Dr. Dwight Lundell is the past Chief of Staff and Chief of Surgery at Banner Heart Hospital, Mesa, AZ. His private practice, Cardiac Care Center was in Mesa, AZ. Recently Dr. Lundell left surgery to focus on the nutritional treatment of heart disease. He is the founder of Healthy Humans Foundation that promotes human health with a focus on helping large corporations promote wellness. He is also the author of The Cure for Heart Disease and The Great Cholesterol Lie.

We physicians with all our training, knowledge and authority often acquire a rather large ego that tends to make it difficult to admit we are wrong. So, here it is. I freely admit to being wrong.. As a heart surgeon with 25 years experience, having performed over 5,000 open-heart surgeries, today is my day to right the wrong with medical and scientific fact.

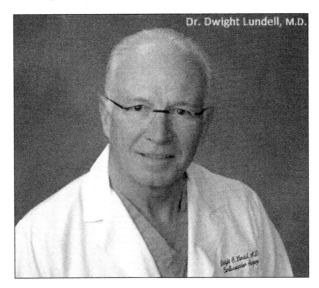

I trained for many years with other prominent physicians labelled "opinion makers." Bombarded with scientific literature, continually attending education seminars, we opinion makers insisted heart disease resulted from the simple fact of elevated blood cholesterol.

The only accepted therapy was prescribing medications to lower cholesterol and a diet that severely restricted fat intake. The latter of course we insisted would lower cholesterol and heart disease. Deviations from these recommendations were considered heresy and could quite possibly result in malpractice.

It Is Not Working!

These recommendations are no longer scientifically or morally defensible. The discovery a few years ago that **inflammation in the artery wall** is the real cause of heart disease is slowing leading to a paradigm shift in how heart disease and other chronic ailments will be treated.

The long-established dietary recommendations have **created epidemics of obesity and diabetes,** the consequences of which dwarf any historical plague in terms of mortality, human suffering and dire economic consequences.

Despite the fact that 25% of the population takes expensive statin medications and despite the fact we have reduced the fat content of our diets, more Americans will die this year of heart disease than ever before.

Statistics from the American Heart Association show that 75 million Americans currently suffer from heart disease, 20 million have diabetes and 57 million have pre-diabetes. These disorders are affecting younger and younger people in greater numbers every year.

Simply stated, without inflammation being present in the body, there is no way that cholesterol would accumulate in the wall of the blood vessel and cause heart disease and strokes. Without inflammation, cholesterol would move freely throughout the body as nature intended. It is inflammation that causes cholesterol to become trapped.

Inflammation is not complicated – it is quite simple your body's natural defence to a foreign invader such as a bacteria, toxin or virus. The cycle of inflammation is perfect in how it protects your body from these bacterial and viral invaders. However, if we **chronically expose the body to injury by toxins or foods the human body was never designed to process, a condition occurs called chronic inflammation.** Chronic inflammation is just as harmful as acute inflammation is beneficial.

What thoughtful person would willfully expose himself repeatedly to foods or other substances that are known to cause injury to the body? Well, smokers perhaps, but at least they made that choice willfully.

The rest of us have simply followed the recommended mainstream diet that is low in fat and high in polyunsaturated fats and carbohydrates, not knowing we were causing repeated injury to our blood vessels. This **repeated injury creates chronic inflammation leading to heart disease, stroke, diabetes and obesity.**

Let me repeat that: **The injury and inflammation in our blood vessels is caused by the low fat diet recommended for years by mainstream medicine.**

What are the biggest culprits of chronic inflammation? Quite simply, they are the overload of simple, highly processed carbohydrates (**sugar, flour** and all the products made from them) and the excess consumption of omega-6 **vegetable oils like soybean, corn and sunflower** that are found in many processed foods.

Take a moment to visualize rubbing a stiff brush repeatedly over soft skin until it becomes quite red and nearly bleeding, you kept this up several times a day, every day for five years. If you could tolerate this painful brushing, you would have a bleeding, swollen infected area that became worse with each repeated injury. This is a good way to visualize the inflammation process that could be going on in your body right now.

Regardless of where the inflammatory process occurs, externally, it is the same. I have peered inside thousands upon thousands of arteries. A diseased artery looks as if someone took a brush and scrubbed repeatedly against its wall. Several times a day, every day, the foods we eat create small injuries compounding into more injuries, causing the body to respond continuously and appropriately with inflammation.

While we savor the tantalizing taste of a sweet roll, our bodies respond alarmingly as if a foreign invader arrived declaring war. **Foods loaded with sugars and simple carbohydrates, or**

processed with omega-6 oils for long shelf life have been the mainstay of the American diet for six decades. These foods have been **slowly poisoning everyone.**

How does eating a simple sweet roll create a cascade of inflammation to make you sick?

Imagine spilling syrup on your keyboard and you have a visual of what occurs inside the cell. When we consume simply carbohydrates such as sugar, blood sugar rises rapidly. In response, your pancreas secretes insulin whose primary purpose is to drive sugar into each cell where it is stored for energy. If the cell is full and does not need glucose, it is rejected to avoid extra sugar gumming up the works.

When your full cells reject the extra glucose, blood sugar rises producing more insulin and the glucose converts to stored fat.

What does all this have to do with inflammation? Blood sugar is controlled in a very narrow range. Extra sugar molecules attach to a variety of proteins that in turn injure the blood vessel wall. This repeated injury to the blood vessel wall sets off inflammation. When you spike your blood sugar level several times a day, every day, it is exactly like taking sandpaper to the inside of your delicate blood vessels.

While you may not be able to see it, rest assured it is there. I saw it in over 5,000 surgical patients spanning 25 years who all shared one common denominator – inflammation in their arteries.

Let's get back to the sweet roll. That innocent looking goody not only contains sugars, it is baked in one of many omega-6 oils such as soybean. Chips and fries are soaked in soybean oil; processed foods are manufactured with omega-6 oils for longer shelf life. While omega-6's are essential – they are part of every cell membrane controlling what goes in and out of the cell – **they must be in the correct balance with omega-3's.**

If the balance shifts by consuming excessive omega-6, the cell membrane produces chemicals called **cytokines that directly cause inflammation.**

Today's mainstream American diet has produced an extreme imbalance of these two fats. The ratio of imbalance ranges from 15:1 to as high as 30:1 in favor of omega-6. That's a tremendous amount of cytokines causing inflammation. In today's food environment, a 3:1 ratio would be optimal and healthy.

To make matters worse, the excess weight you are carrying from eating these foods creates overloaded fat cells that pour out large quantities of pro-inflammation chemicals that add to the injury caused by having high blood sugar. The process that began with a sweet roll turns into a vicious cycle over time that creates **heart disease, high blood pressure, diabetes** and finally, **Alzheimer's disease,** as the inflammation process continues unabated.

There is but one answer to quieting inflammation, and that is returning to foods closer to their natural state. To build muscle, eat more protein. Choose carbohydrates that are very complex such as **coloring fruits and vegetables.** Cut down on or eliminate inflammation-causing omega-6 fats like corn and soybean oil and the processed foods that are made from them.

One tablespoon of corn oil contains 7,280 mg of omega-6; soybean contains 6,940 mg. Instead, use **olive oil or butter from** grass-fed beef.

Animals fats contain less than 20% omega-6 and are much less likely to cause inflammation than the supposedly healthy oils labeled polyunsaturated. Forget the "science" that has been drummed into your head for decades. The science that saturated fat alone causes heart disease is non-existent. The science that saturated fat raises blood cholesterol is also very weak. Since we now know that cholesterol is not the cause of heart disease, the concern about saturated fat is even more absurd today.

The cholesterol theory led to the no-fat, low-fat recommendations that in turn created the very foods now causing an epidemic of inflammation. Mainstream medicine made a terrible mistake when it advised people to avoid saturated fat in favor of foods high in omega-6 fats. We now have an epidemic of arterial inflammation leading to heart disease and other silent killers.

What you can do is choose **whole foods** your grandmother served and not those your mom turned to as grocery store aisles filled with manufactured foods. By eliminating inflammation foods and adding essential nutrients from **fresh unprocessed food,** you will reverse years of damage in your arteries and throughout your body from consuming the typical American diet.

John 8:32 says, "And ye shall know the truth, and the truth shall make you free."

What is inflammation?

Inflammation is the first response of the immune system to infection or irritation. We are all familiar with the classic signs of inflammation (swelling, redness and pain) that occur when we hurt ourselves or have some kind of infection. However recent research[1] has shown that eating the wrong foods can cause inflammation within our bodies. In fact being overweight can itself be the cause of inflammation.

Body fat causes inflammation

The fatty tissues of the body secrete hormones that regulate the immune system and inflammation, but in the case of an overweight individual this can become out of control. Three of the hormones that play a role in metabolism are leptin, resistin and adiponectin.

- Leptin is involved in appetite control.
- Resistin is a hormone that increases insulin resistance.
- Adiponectin lowers the blood sugar by making your body more insulin sensitive.

The fact that it is the fatty tissue that produces these hormones makes the fat self regulating, as the hormones should act to bring the increased fat under control. Bodies with more fat will produce more leptin bringing the appetite under control. However in cases where the body is inflamed there is often a problem with leptin resistance, and the self regulation of fat does not occur. Leptin resistance is where to body stops responding to the appetite controlling effects of the hormone.

In addition to these metabolism regulating hormones your fatty tissue also produces chemicals that cause inflammation and this can make the problem of leptin resistance worse. This is why obesity can cause an increase of these inflammatory chemicals which in turn inhibit the correct balancing function of the weight controlling hormones. This results in a vicious circle of weight gain causing inflammation which inhibits hormone function thereby causing further weight gain.

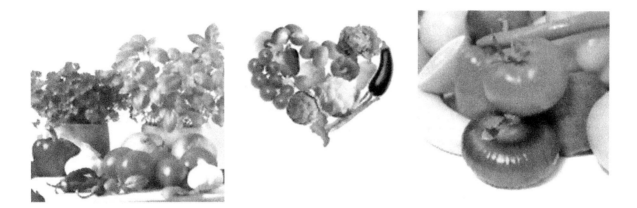

Genesis 1:11, 12 says, "And God said, Let the earth bring forth grass, the herb yielding seed, and the fruit tree yielding fruit after his kind, whose seed is in itself, upon the earth: and it was so. And the earth brought forth grass, and herb yielding seed after his kind, and the tree yielding fruit, whose seed was in itself, after his kind: and God saw that it was good."

Genesis 1:29 says, "And God said, Behold, I have given you every herb bearing seed, which is upon the face of all the earth, and every tree, in the which is the fruit of a tree yielding seed; to you it shall be for meat."

"Chase after the truth like hell and you will free yourself even though you never touch its coat tails."

Clarence Seward Darrow

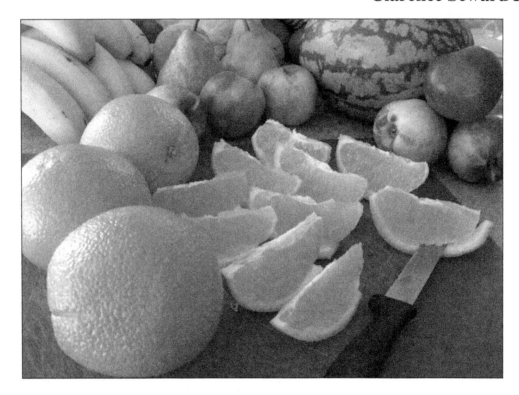

...Dominion, God blessed man by letting him have dominion over every living thing that moveth upon the earth. Genesis 1:28.

Fruits and vegetables are indeed living things and according to Genesis 1:29, they shall be for meat.

Eight Foods You Should Almost Never, Ever Eat.

Most soybean, corn, cotton and canola crops in the U.S. are genetically altered. Some experts argue that these crops could pose serious health and environmental risks, but the scientific picture is currently incomplete -- deliberately so.

Agricultural corporations such as Monsanto and Syngenta have restricted independent research on the crops. They have refused to provide independent scientists with seeds, or else have set restrictive conditions that severely limit research. This is legal because under U.S. law, genetically engineered crops are patentable.

The Los Angeles Times reports:

> *"Agricultural companies defend their stonewalling by saying that unrestricted research could make them vulnerable to lawsuits if an experiment somehow leads to harm, or that it could give competitors unfair insight into their products. But it's likely that the companies fear something else as well: An experiment could reveal that a genetically engineered product is hazardous or doesn't perform as promised."*

Even if you don't want to eat genetically engineered foods, you most likely already are doing so. Corn and soy are two of the most common food ingredients, especially in processed foods, and over 90 percent of both these crops in the US are now from GM seeds.

Organic food companies and consumer groups are stepping up their efforts to get the government to exercise more oversight of engineered foods. Critics of current policy argue that the genetically modified (GM) seeds are often contaminating the nearby non-GM crops.

ABC News reports:

> *"The U.S. government has insisted there's not enough difference between the genetically modified seeds its agencies have approved and natural seeds to cause concern. But Agriculture Secretary Tom Vilsack, more so than his predecessors in previous administrations, has acknowledged the debate over the issue and a growing chorus of consumers concerned about what they are eating."*

"And ye shall know the truth, and the truth shall make you free."

St. John 8:32

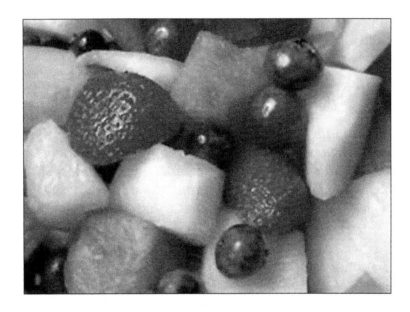

Proverbs 9:6 says, "Forsake the foolish, and live; and go in the way of understanding."

God's natural seeded water melons

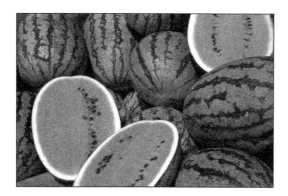

Numbers 11:5 says, "We remember the fish, which we did eat in Egypt freely; the cucumbers, and the melons, and the leeks, and the onions, and the garlic;"

The Watermelon You Should Never, Ever Eat
Posted By Dr. Mercola | June 03 2011

Watermelon fields in eastern China are covered in exploded fruit. Farmers used growth chemicals to make their crops bigger, but ended up destroying them instead.

The farmers used the growth accelerator forchlorfenuron. Even the melons that survived tended to have fibrous, misshapen fruit with mostly white instead of black seeds.

MSNBC reports:

"Chinese regulations don't forbid use of the substance. It is also allowed in the United States for use on kiwi fruit and grapes... About 20 farmers and 115 acres of watermelon around Danyang were affected... Farmers resorted to chopping up the fruit and feeding it to fish and pigs".

What is Forchlorfenuron?

Forchlorfenuron is a so-called "plant growth regulator," registered with the US Environmental Protection Agency (EPA) in 2004 for use on grapes, raisins, and kiwis. According to the EPA Pesticide Fact sheet, the chemical is to be applied to the flowers and/or developing fruit during early post-bloom to improve fruit size, fruit set, cluster weight, and cold storage. The fact sheet explains that the chemical "acts synergistically with natural auxins to promote plant cell division and lateral growth."

According to MSNBC, the Chinese farmers incorrectly applied forchlorfenuron to the fruit "during overly wet weather and... too late in the season, which made the melons burst."

Indeed. Melons have been exploding by the acre.

Another article published on May 24 by The Epoch Times, specified that the seeds used were "quality watermelon seeds" imported from Japan. Of the 20 farmers in the affected Chinese province, 10 of them used these imported Japanese seeds. It's unclear whether all of the farmers whose crops blew up had also used forchlorfenuron.

But ruptured melon-heads are not the most concerning aspect of this story. There's also the question of consumer safety. Although no specific health hazards are mentioned in any of the articles covering this story, they do allude to the fact that there may be cause for health concerns.

Are Growth Promoting Chemicals Safe to Eat?

MSNBC writes:

"The report quoted Feng Shuangqing, a professor at the China Agricultural University, as saying the problem showed that China needs to clarify its farm chemical standards and supervision to protect consumer health. the report underscores how farmers in China are abusing both legal and illegal chemicals, with many farms misusing pesticides and fertilizers."

Forchlorfenuron is in fact legal, both in China and in the US. But should it be? According to the EPA pesticide fact sheet, forchlorfenuron is not necessarily harmless, neither to the environment nor to animals and potentially humans. Side effects revealed in animal studies included:

- Increased incidence of alopecia (hair loss)
- Decreased birth weight
- Increased pup mortality
- Decreased litter sizes

They also categorize forchlorfenuron as "moderately toxic to freshwater fish on an acute basis."

How to Spot Fruit Grown with Growth Accelerating Chemicals

One of the tell-tale signs of a fruit or vegetable that hasn't been grown by entirely natural means is their inherent *lack of flavor*. It may look plump and ripe, but once you bite into it, it's anything but a flavor sensation. This is because while growth enhancers like forchlorfenuron stimulate cell division, making the fruit grow faster, it also drains it of flavor. This is actually rather logical, if you think about it. Flavor is a sign of ripeness, which only comes with time. Many unripe fruits and vegetables are virtually tasteless.

In the case of watermelons, those treated with forchlorfenuron are very large and brightly colored on the outside, but the color of the flesh is more white than deep red. Other telltale signs are white instead of black seeds and fibrous, and/or misshapen fruit. (Note, this is for regular watermelons, which have black seeds. Seedless watermelons typically have tiny white seeds.)

Hormones in Your Fruits and Veggies? You Bet!

This is an area that doesn't get much press. While many are now aware of the fact that CAFO raised meats are loaded with hormones, few would imagine that fresh produce would be laced with hormone additives as well. But they are. According to Zheng Fengtian, a professor of agriculture from Renmin University, hormones can increase yields by 20 percent or more, and are therefore "widely used."

Some of these hormones you might never expect to make their way onto your plate, such as oxytocin—a hormone that acts as a neuromodulator in your brain; often referred to as "the love hormone," or "bonding hormone." It's released naturally in large amounts in a woman's body during childbirth, but has also been synthesized biochemically and is available as a prescription drug to induce labor—and is, apparently, being illegally injected into fruits and vegetables in some countries...

Last summer, an <u>Indian health minister, Dinesh Trivedi, warned about the illegal use of oxytocin in fruits</u> and vegetables in India. Apparently the hormone allows produce to gain weight and ripen sooner. Injected produce also appear plumper and fresher.

According to Trivedi, the hormone is being used on:

- Pumpkins
- Watermelons

- Cucumbers
- Aubergines

FoodSafety.com also reported that the drug, although banned for public sale in India, was widely available from fertilizer and pesticide vendors. Potential side effects of consuming oxytocin-laced produce include:

| Irregular heartbeat | Nausea | Vomiting | Cramping |
| Stomach pain | Sterility | Neurotic complications | Nervous breakdowns |

Other Growth Promoters Used on Produce

Other growth promoting agents used in fruits and vegetables include:

- Ethylene (used to ripen mangoes)
- Calcium carbide (used on apples, papayas, and guavas)

While ethylene is considered GRAS (generally recognized as safe), calcium carbide "may contain traces of arsenic and phosphorus, both highly toxic to humans," according to one industry source, and most countries do not allow its use.

Interestingly enough, one of the Chinese farmers whose melons exploded reportedly used a formula containing a mixture of growth enhancers, sweetening agents, and "a calcium solution." So it's not clear whether the formula used on the exploding fruits contained calcium carbide in conjunction with the forchlorfenuron. Whatever the case may be, the results are clearly not good.

Still on the Fence about Going Organic?

If you're still vacillating on the issue of going organic, I hope this information spurs you into action.

If you eat conventionally grown produce, not only are you exposing yourself and your family to a variety of pesticides; you may also get hormones and chemical growth promoters—all of which have the potential to devastate your health, especially that of young children. Remember, conventional produce sold in your local supermarket comes from all over the world! So you cannot brush off this information as being a potential threat affecting just the region in which the produce was grown.

Organic foods also contain higher amounts of nutrients, so you're getting "more bang for your buck," when seen from a nutrition standpoint. One four-year long European-Union-funded study found that:

- Organic fruit and vegetables contain up to 40 percent more antioxidants
- Organic produce had higher levels of beneficial minerals like iron and zinc
- Milk from organic herds contained up to 90 percent more antioxidants

Last but not least, if you're any kind of food aficionado, meaning if you *like flavor*, organic foods simply cannot be beat. When it comes to produce, your absolute best bet is *locally-grown organics*. That's truly the best of both worlds. However, if you can't find locally grown organics, opt for USDA certified organic, but not imported organic, over the conventionally grown variety. Just be aware that wilted organic produce is not going to provide the nutrition that a fresh one will, even if it's conventionally grown, so freshness is also key.

There are some exceptions to the all-organic rule, which may be welcome news if you cannot afford to buy everything organic. For more information on which conventionally-grown produce are the safest, please see my previous article 12 Foods You Don't Have to Buy Organic.

Pay Now, or Pay Later...

My personal view of why you'd want an organic lifestyle is that although you may spend more money on organic food today, your payoff of good health should more than make up for it – and reduce your health care costs in the future. It makes sense to me to invest a little bit more now so I can avoid paying LARGE medical bills later on, but more importantly, I can avoid the physical and mental disability and dysfunction that inevitably follows from a careless, unhealthy lifestyle. Making sure you're not being misled by labels in your search for a healthier lifestyle is unfortunately part of this process. However, by educating yourself about what to look for, talking to your grocer, and sharing information with family, friends and neighbors, you can help the movement toward healthier food choices.

Also Beware of Genetically Modified Foods

Buying organic will also help you avoid yet another major health hazard in our food supply, namely genetically modified (GM) foods. I strongly recommend looking for foods that are "non-GMO certified" by the Non-GMO Project. For your convenience, download this Non-GMO Shopping Guide, and share it with everyone you know.

Although GM foods still do not require labeling by law, the campaign for GMO labeling is making progress, thanks to the persistence of Jeffrey Smith and the Institute for Responsible Technology, an organization whose goal is to end the genetic engineering of our food supply and the outdoor release of GM crops. If you like, you can join the fight by signing the petition to President Obama in support of mandatory labeling of GM foods.

For ongoing updates on this cause, please follow our Non-GMO's page on Facebook.

By educating the public about the risks of GM foods through a massive education campaign, and by circulating the Non-GMO Shopping Guide so consumers can make healthier non-GMO choices, the Institute's plan is to generate a tipping point of consumer rejection to make GMOs a thing of the past.

Remember food is a critical part of the equation of "Taking Control of Your Health", you simply must get it right if you want any real chance of avoiding chronic degenerative disease.

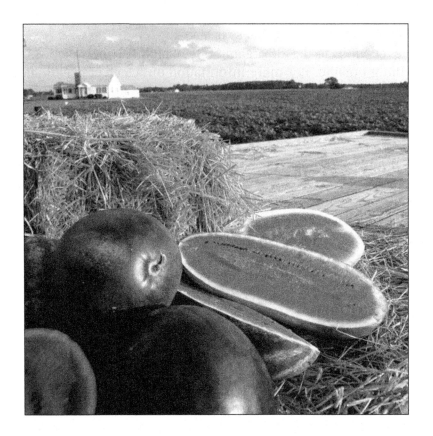

The seeded crops of today's watermelon harvest sets the stage for next year's harvest and watermelon harvest for generations to come.

Genesis 1:11 says, "And God said, Let the earth bring forth grass, the herb yielding seed, and the fruit tree yielding fruit after his kind, whose seed is in itself, upon the earth: and it was so."

Numbers 11:5 says, "We remember the fish, which we did eat in Egypt freely; the cucumbers, and the melons, and the leeks, and the onions, and the garlic;"

Wild Natural Garlic

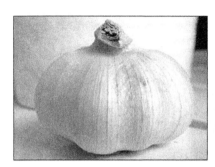 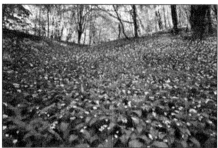

Numbers 11:5 says, "We remember the fish, which we did eat in Egypt freely; the cucumbers, and the melons, and the leeks, and the onions, and the garlic;"

"…and by the river upon the bank thereof, shall grow all tree for meat, and the fruit therefore shall be for meat, and the leaf thereof for medicine."

Ezekiel 47:12

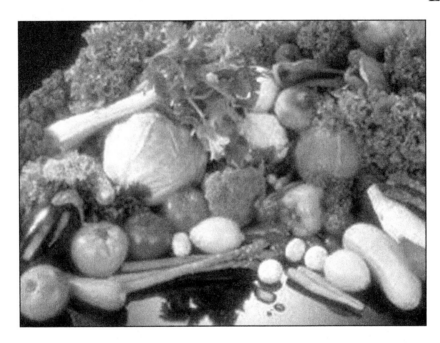

John 8:32 says, "And ye shall know the truth, and the truth shall make you free."

CDC, Center for Disease Control

These are my tables; according to the CDC, Center for Disease Control and Prevention and the National Center for Health Statistics, of the top ten causes of death in the United States, the first four are all food borne diseases with the fifth cause of death being; Accidents (unintentional injuries). The remaining causes of death of the top ten causes of death are food borne diseases as well. These diseases are based on a violation of God's Principles. See below;

Leading Causes of Death 2007

(Data are for the U.S.), CDC Center for Disease Control & Prevention

National Center for Health Statistics

Number of deaths for leading causes of death

• • • Top ten causes of death 9 are food borne diseases.

- Heart disease: 616,067
- Cancer: 562,875
- Stroke (cerebrovascular diseases): 135,952
- Chronic lower respiratory diseases: 127,924
- Accidents (unintentional injuries): 123,706
- Alzheimer's disease: 74,632
- Diabetes: 71,382
- Influenza and Pneumonia: 52,717
- Nephritis, nephrotic syndrome, and nephrosis: 46,448
- Septicemia: 34,828

Wild Locust

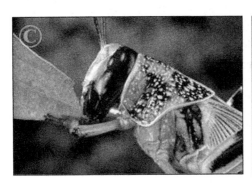 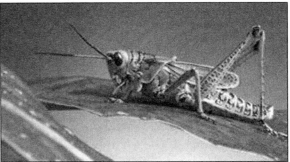

St. Mark 1:6 says, "And John was clothed with camel's hair, and with a girdle of a skin about his loins; and he did eat locusts and wild honey;"

DID YOU KNOW?

Article #3: Black Pepper Causes Cancer!

Confirmation of Life Science's teaching that anything taken into the body that is not a food is poisonous and harmful comes from the research laboratory of the University of Kentucky.

Life Science teaches not to use condiments on, in or with our foods—or by themselves. In fact, we teach to eat only foods that are a gustatory delight in themselves. For good health we must eat only those foods that don't call for the addition of seasonings or spices of any sort. Foods and so-called foods that have to be jazzed up with condiments are unhealthful.

When black pepper was given to mice at the University of Kentucky, they developed problems aplenty, including cancer of the liver, lungs and skin. This is a prime example of how toxic processed condiments really are. Cayenne pepper, chili powder, salt, basil, cumin seed, caraway, vinegar, processed garlic and hundreds of other condiments (herbs, seasonings, spices) are likewise pathogenic and carcinogenic.

To attain and maintain health, you need to drop condiments from your life—forever. Eat only fresh raw succulent fruits, vegetables, nuts, seeds and sprouts. The better your diet, the better you'll look and feel.

Reprinted from Health Crusader April 1980

Suggested cooking temperatures for meat.

Meat Temperature Chart

The **US Department of Agriculture** says the following temperatures will produce safely cooked, but still flavorful* meats:

Meat	Internal Temp.	Centigrade
Fresh ground beef, veal, lamb, pork	160°F	71°C
Beef, veal, lamb roasts, steaks, chops: medium rare	145°F	63°C
Beef, veal, lamb roasts, steaks, chops: medium	160°F	71°C
Beef, veal, lamb roasts, steaks, chops: well done	170°F	77°C
Fresh pork roasts, steaks, chops: medium	160°F	71°C
Fresh pork roasts, steaks, chops: well done	170°F	77°C
Ham: cooked before eating	160°F	71°C
Ham: fully cooked, to reheat	140°F	60°C
Ground chicken/turkey	165°F	74°C
Whole chicken/turkey	180°F	82°C
Poultry breasts, roasts	170°F	77°C

* Not everyone agrees with the US Department of Agriculture.

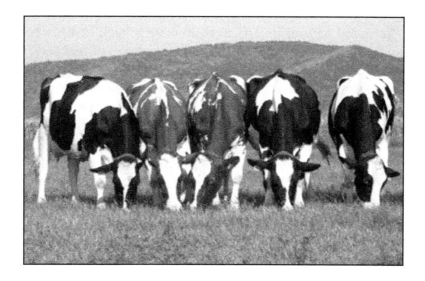

- **Psalms 104:14** says, "He causeth the grass to grow for the cattle, and herb for the service of man: that he may bring forth food out of the earth;"

- **Deuteronomy 11:15** says, "And I will send grass in thy fields for thy cattle, that thou mayest eat and be full."

100% Grass-Fed Natural Beef

Nutritional Analysis

Slanker's 100% grass-fed natural beef is a positive step back in time because it gives consumers the old-fashioned flavor and natural nutritional advantages of real beef. Better flavor makes dining more enjoyable. Better nutrition improves health and fitness, which increases self-esteem, peace of mind, and long term security.

Sometimes folks ask for a nutritional analysis of grass-fed meats. Well, a complete analysis would be so extensive it would be beyond the known needs of animal life! Since we know the green leaf is the foundation food for all animal life, the nutrients in grass-fed meats and their relative balance are down the centerline for the nutrient requirements our human bodies require – no more no less. There is no other food that compares to the nutritional perfection of meat from a grass-fed critter. Therefore, grass-fed meats are a nutrient standard.

It wasn't until after man started eating grain, grain-based foods, and grain-fed livestock did he start to worry about the nutritional analysis of his anemic foods. That's when he discovered he had to also invent nutritional supplements. Grass –fed meats are not anemic. Consequently one just eats them like man did prior to inventing grain farming and the concocting of foods. Therefore we do not worry about measuring. We just eat. (See The Real Diet of Man is Very Simple.) Check out the abbreviated nutritional ledger below. Note how grain feeding drastically lowers vitamin levels and skews fatty acid profiles in just this short list of selected nutrients. If grain does that to cattle, it also does that to people.

Beef's Nutritional Ledger		
	Grain-Fed Beef	**Grass-Fed Beef**
Added Hormones	Usually	No
Fed Antibiodics	Usually	No
Fed Grain	Yes	No
Omega-3 Fatty Acids	0.10	1.22
Omega-6 Fatty Acids	3.10	1.08
CLA	0.21	1.46
Beta Carotene	41.00	87.00
Vitamin E	1.30	5.30
Vitamin A	10.00	52.00
Total Fat	High & Saturated	Perfect Balance
Flavor	Bland/Pasty	Original and Bold
All Other Factors	Fair	Perfect
E. Coli Risk	Present	Not Likely

With 100% grass-fed beef consumers are rediscovering the real meaty flavor beef always had prior to the "invention" of the feedlot. With 50% less saturated fat grass-fed beef does not feel greasy because it isn't greasy. Nor does grass-fed beef leave a pasty tasting, greasy feeling in your mouth when you eat it.

Nutritional scientists report that by switching to grass-fed beef you will lose weight, have a healthier heart, reduce your risk of cancer, diabetes, arthritis, and allergies, improve mental clarity, and more.

These health claims sound almost too good to be true, yet the scientific evidence is overwhelming. The reasons involve fundamental nutritional differences. Compared to grain-fed beef, grass-fed beef has higher levels of Conjugated Linoleic Acid (CLA), more Beta Carotene, more Omega 3 fatty acids, more Vitamins A and E, and lower levels of saturated fats. These attributes and nutrients are essential for good health. Americans must start paying attention to their nutrient intake and reduce their consumption of saturated fats, trans-fatty acids (partially hydrogenated oils), grain-filled processed food products, and grain-fed livestock products. If they don't, health and health care costs will remain their number one concern.

Slanker's Grass-Fed Meats – Ted Slanker
3255 CR 45400, Powerly, Texas 75473
903-732-4653 Office – 866-SLANKER (752-6537) Toll Free
http://texasgrassfedbeef.com/ email at goodmeat@slanker.com

- **Psalms 104:14** He causeth the grass to grow for the cattle, and herb for the service of man: that he may bring forth food out of the earth;

- **Deuteronomy 11:15** And I will send grass in thy fields for thy cattle, that thou mayest eat and be full.

> - **Isaiah 40:6-8** the voice said, Cry. And he said, what shall I cry? <u>All</u> withereth, the flower fadeth: because the spirit of the Lord bloweth upon it: <u>surely the people is grass</u>. The grass withereth, the flower fadeth: but the word of our God shall stand for ever. <u>flesh is grass</u>, and all the goodliness thereof is as the flower of the field: The grass.

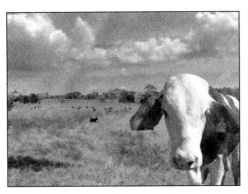 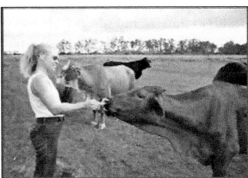

- **Psalms 104:14** says, "He causeth the grass to grow for the cattle, and herb for the service of man: that he may bring forth food out of the earth;"

Warning! Alert! Alert! Human consumption of any meats should be avoided if that animal did not have a natural source of feed.

These fed lot cattle below are being fed food a totally unnatural diet that is against God's principles and instructions. Therefore the fed lot cattle nutritional value is below the nutritional value of God's grass fed cattle according to the Beef's Nutritional Ledger above and countless other nutritional reports.

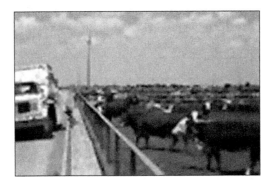

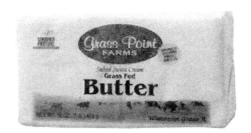

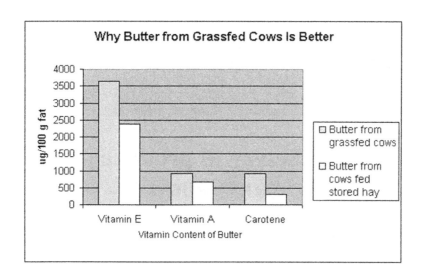

Proverbs 30:33 says, "Surely the churning of milk bringeth foth butter…"

II Samuel 17:29 says, "And honey, and butter, and sheep, and cheese of kine, for David, and for the people that were with him, to eat: for they said, The people is hungry, and weary, and thirsty, in the wilderness."

Tropical Traditions, Inc., PO Box 333, Springville, Ca 93265, 1-559-539-2986

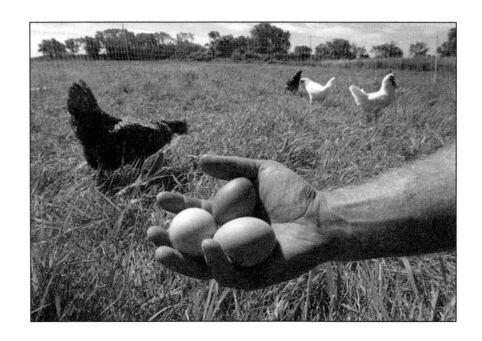

Naturally fed chickens will produce all natural free range eggs.

Isaiah 10:14 says, "And **my hand hath found as a nest** the riches of the people: and as **one gathereth eggs that are left,** have I gathered all the earth; and there was none that moved the wing, or opened the mouth, or peeped."

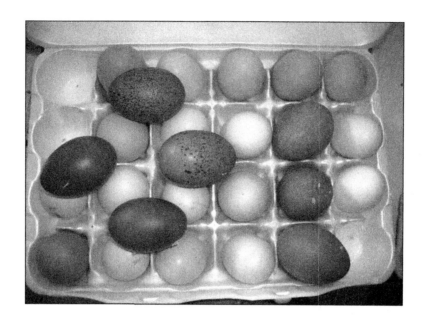

Photo illustrates wide range in God's natural color rendering.

Job 6:6 says, "Can that which is unsavoury be eaten without salt? or is there any taste in the white of an **egg**?"

Luke 11:12 says, "Or if he shall ask an **egg**, will he offer him a scorpion?"

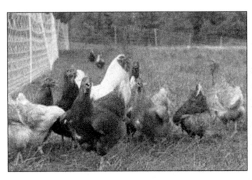
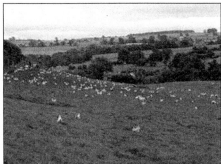

God created chickens, so that makes chickens a natural resource. When natural resources consume food, it would be against **God's** instructions and principles for that food source to be anything other than natural sources. When the chickens have access to **God's** open range, then they will follow **God's instructions** and eat that which **God has made available for them to eat.** Free range chickens are indeed a natural of protein supplied by our **heavenly Father**.

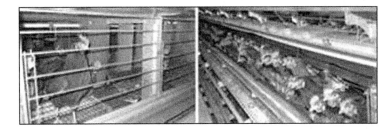

Warning! Human consumption of any meats should be avoided if that animal did not have a natural source of feed.

Caged chickens have no access to **God's** natural feed resources.

God's Basket

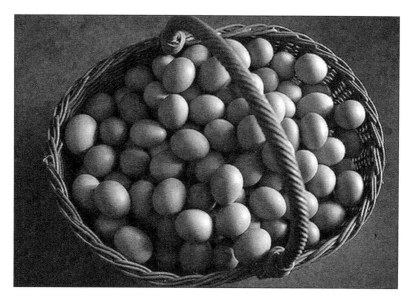

It's been said that man should never put all of his eggs in one basket.

Hebrews 11:1, 2, 3 says, "NOW FAITH is the substance of things hoped for, the evidence of things not seen. For by it the elders obtained a good report. Through faith we understand that the worlds were framed by the word of God, so that things which are seen were not made of things which do appear."

Hebrews 11: 5, 6 says, "By faith Enoch was translated that he should not see death …for before his translation he had this testimony, that he pleased God. But without faith it is impossible to please him: for he that cometh to God must believe that he is, and that he is a rewarder of them that diligently seek him."

Please God, stay faithful, put all of your eggs in God's basket.

Grass-Fed Lamb

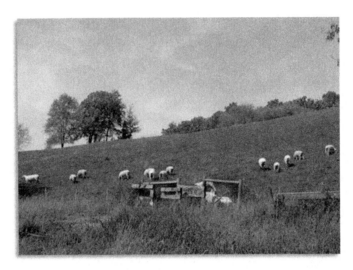

100% Grass-fed Lamb!

Grass-Fed Traditions supplies 100% grass-fed lamb from small-scale family farms in Wisconsin. These sheep graze on lush pasture all summer long in the rolling hills of the "Driftless Area" of southwestern Wisconsin. The Driftless Area of Wisconsin is famous around the world because it is completely surrounded by glaciated territory. It preserves a large sample of what the rest of Wisconsin, as well as northern and eastern United States, were like before the Glacial Period. The Driftless Area is driftless because of three factors: 1. The highland to the north furnished temporary protection from ice invasion. 2. The more rapid movement of glacial lobes in the lowland to the east and the region to the west resulted in the final joining of these ice lobes south of the Driftless Area, so that it was completely surrounded by the continental glacier. 3. The termination of the forward movement and the beginning of retreat came before there was time for the ice from the north, east and west to cover the driftless remnant. The result is a unique geographical area of rolling hills that the early settlers of Wisconsin recognized was especially well-suited for grazing. Today many small-scale family farms still graze this rich soil, and some of the most world-renown artisan cheeses are also from this rich agricultural area of Wisconsin. **Grass-Fed Traditions** now offers premium grass-fed lamb grazed on pastures from this same rich soil of Wisconsin. We believe you will not find tastier lamb from anywhere in the world!

How do we define "grass-fed?" The sheep are on pasture, not in feed lots eating silage. They are also finished on grass, and do not eat grains at all. We don't process animals in the winter or early spring, when they are only eating dry grass. Our animals are eating green grass right up to the time of processing. All of our pastures are free from the use of pesticides or other chemical treatments, and completely organic.

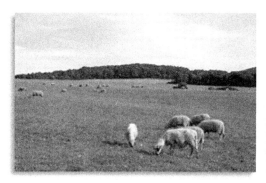 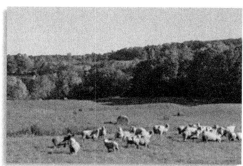

Conjugated Linoleic Acid (CLA) is a naturally occurring free fatty acid found mainly in meat and dairy products in small amounts. CLA was discovered by accident in 1978 by Michael W. Pariza at the University of Wisconsin while looking for mutagen formations in meat during cooking. The most abundant source of natural CLA is the meat and dairy products of grass-fed animals. Research conducted since 1999 shows that grazing animals have from 3-5 times more CLA than animals fattened on grain in a feedlot. Simply switching from grain-fed to grass-fed products can greatly increase your intake of CLA. (Dhiman, T. R., G. R. Anand, et al. (1999). "Conjugated linoleic acid content of milk from cows fed different diets." J Dairy Sci 82(10): 2146-56

Omega 3 is an essential fatty acid for human growth and development. We must have it to be healthy. Grass-finished lamb is a great source for this essential nutrient. The source of Omega 3 is the green leaves of plants. When sheep eat their natural diet, lamb becomes a great source of Omega 3. Grain is not a rich source of Omega 3, so standard, grain-finishing practices cause the Omega 3 level to decrease dramatically.

Tropical Traditions, Inc., PO Box 333, Springville, Ca 93265, Corporate Office: West Bend, WI 53095, http://www.tropicaltraditions.com/ Founders, Brian & Marianita Shilhavy 1-559-539-2986

Grass Fed Goats

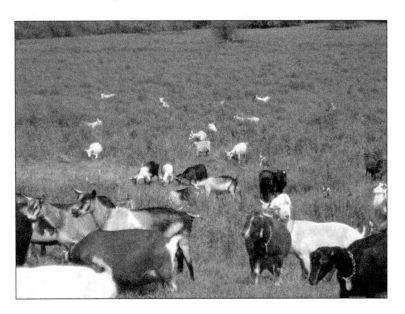

Genesis 27:9,10 says, "Go now to the flock, and fetch me from thence two good kids of the goats; and I will make them savoury meat for thy father, such as he loveth: And thou shalt bring it to thy father, that he may eat, and that he may bless thee before his death."

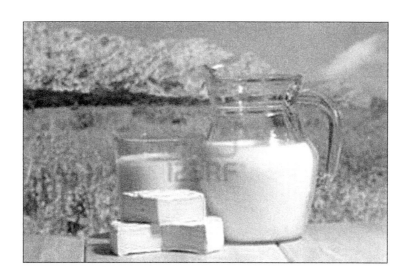

Goat's milk and cheese

Proverbs 27:27 says, "And thou shalt have goats milk enough for thy food, for the food of thy household, and for the maintenance for thy maidens."

White Tail Deer

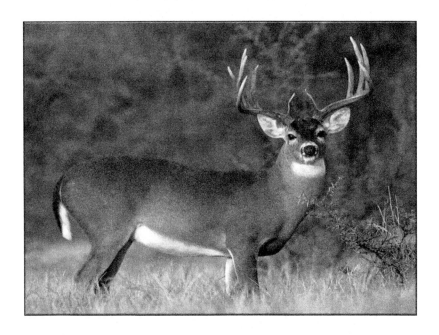

Genesis 27:7 says, **"Bring me venison, and make me savoury meat, that I may eat, and bless thee before the Lord before my death."**

Wild Turkeys

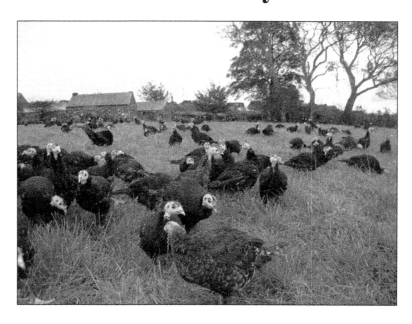

Photo of, feeding free range organic turkeys, God's work.

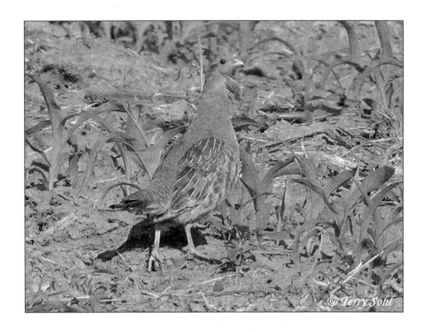

Gray Partridge

1 Samuel 26:20 says, "Now therefore, let not my blood fall to the earth before the face of the Lord: for the king of Israel is come out to seek a flea, as when one doth hunt a partridge in the mountains."

Wild caught fish from God's all natural rare earth are the most nutritious for human consumption and bears as well.

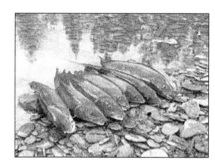 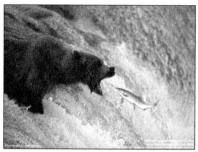

Matthew 15:36 says, "And he took the seven loaves and the fishes, and gave thanks, and brake, them, and gave to his disciples, and the disciples to the multitude."

Number 11:5 says, "We remember the fish, which we did eat in Egypt freely; the cucumbers, and the melons, and the leeks, and the onions, and the garlic:"

Farmed fish are fed a diet that is not natural by man and the food industry and should be avoided.

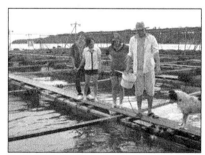 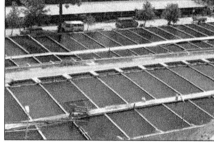

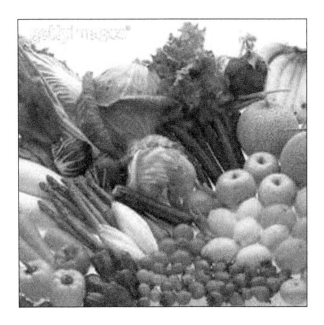

Joshua 5:12 says, "And the manna ceased on the morrow after they had eaten of the old corn of the land; neither had the children of Israel manna any more; but they did eat of the fruit of the land of Canaan that year."

Ezekiel 25:4 says, "Behold, therefore I will deliver thee to the men of the east for a possession, and they shall set their palaces in thee, and make their dwellings in thee: they shall eat thy fruit, and they shall drink thy milk."

All Natural Almond Trees

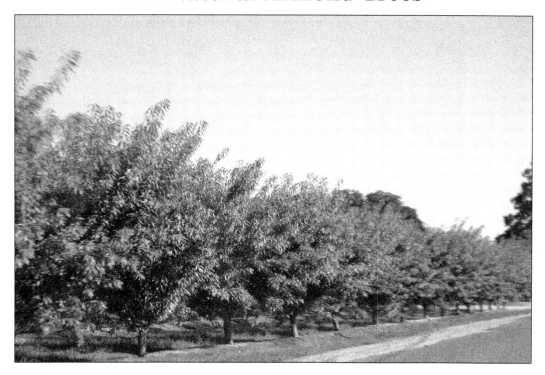

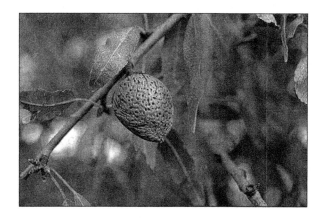

All Natural Almonds

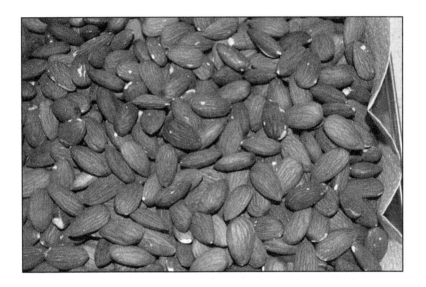

Genesis 43:11 says, "And their father Israel said unto them, if it must be so now, do this; take of the best fruits in the land in your vessels, and carry down the man a present, a little balm, and a little honey, spices, and myrrh, nuts, and almonds:"

Numbers 17:8 says, "And it came to pass, that on the morrow Moses went into the tabernacle of witness; and, behold, the rod of Aaron for the house of Levi was budded, and brought forth buds, and bloomed blossoms, and yielded almonds."

All Natural Cucumbers

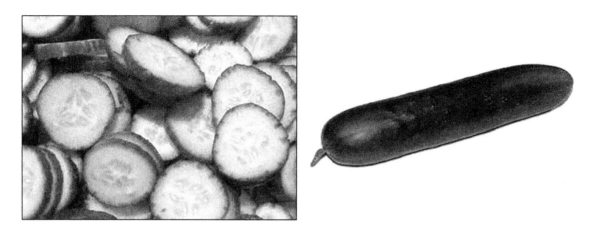

Numbers 11:5 says, "We remember the fish, which we did eat in Egypt freely; the cucumbers, and the melons, and the leeks, and the onions, and the garlic;"

CHAIN OF LIFE, ENZYMES

The key is to remember that <u>food enzymes are destroyed at temperatures above **118 F.**</u> This means that cooked and processed foods contain few, if any enzymes, and that the typical North American diet is enzyme-deficient. When we eat this type of diet, we could well be eating for a shorter and less-than-healthy life.

THE FOOD CHAIN OR ECOSYSTEM AND LIFE CYCLES FOR ANIMALS

This ecosystem consists of four parts. It begins with the sun at the top, which provides energy to our green plants. Green plants such as grass uses the sun to produce sugar and protein in order to grow. The ecosystem consists of producers and consumers. Plants are producers in the ecosystem chain. Animals, which are consumers, are next in the ecosystem. Some of these animals are known as herbivores, which only eat plants. Carnivores are the animals that get their energy from eating other animals. The next categories are the people and animals that eat plants and animals, which are omnivores. The ecosystem described herein is not a man made system. The all mighty creator created all of the components of this ecosystem; hence we live in an all-natural finely tuned divine ecosystem. The system works when all of God's principles are honored and applied.

When any of the components are modified or changed by man, then the system is no longer natural.

- **Genesis 1:26** And God said, Let us make man in our image, after our likeness…

This verse leads us to believe that man is a natural creation. As a natural creation, man needs to consume natural foods or fuels in order to live a natural life free of disease. We must guard against over cooking the food or fuel we eat. Food should be prepared with the intent of not destroying the enzymes. **The enzymes in the food we eat must expire in your digestive system.**

This is important to remember. Dr. Edward Howell, who has written two books on enzymes, theorizes that humans are given a limited supply of enzyme energy at birth, and that it is up to us to replenish our supply of enzymes to ensure that their vital jobs get done. If we don't replenish our supply, we run the risk of ill health.

In the Enzyme Nutrition axiom, Howell postulates, "The length of life is inversely proportional to the rate of exhaustion of the enzyme potential of an organism. The increased use of food enzymes promotes a decreased rate of exhaustion of the enzyme potential."

In other words, the more food enzymes you get, the longer, and healthier, you live.

Wild Organic Honey

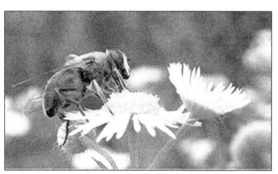 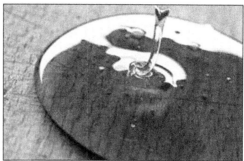

Genesis 43:11 says, "And their father Israel said unto them, if it must be so now, do this; take of the best fruits in the land in your vessels, and carry down the man a present, a little balm, and a little honey, spices, and myrrh, nuts, and almonds:"

II Samuel 17:29 says, "And honey, and butter, and sheep, and cheese of kine, for David, and for the people that were with him, to eat: for they said, The people is hungry, and weary, and thirsty, in the wilderness."

All Natural Stevia

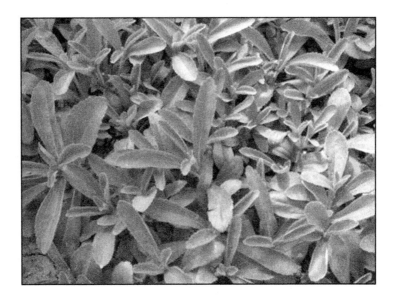

Stevia is an all natural sugar replacement that does not have a glycemic load and measures zero on the glycemic index.

What are the Benefits of Stevia?

A number of studies show that Stevia can be beneficial in the treatment of many health conditions. Stevia is believed to have anti-bacterial, anti-septic, anti-microbial, anti-oxidant, anti-glycemic, and anti-hypertensive properties which may help with hypertension (high blood pressure), diabetes, chronic fatigue, indigestion, upset stomach, heartburn, weight loss, cold and flu, gingivitis, tooth decay, cavities, dandruff and hair loss, brittle bones or osteoporosis, streptococcus, candidiasis, bacterial infections and skin conditions such as cuts, wounds, rashes, itchiness, blemishes, acne, seborrhoeic dermatitis, dermatitis, eczema, and wrinkles. It may also improve energy levels, strengthen immune system, stimulate mental activity, and may also help in withdrawl from tobacco and alcohol addiction.

Uses of Stevia

Dandruff and Hair Health

Stevia concentrate is believed to be beneficial for dandruff, dry scalp, and dull, dry and thin hair. People have noticed stronger, dandruff-free and rejuvenated hair after the regular use of Stevia. Simply mix 3-4 drops of Stevia concentrate into your regular shampoo and wash as normal. Also, after shampooing, using stevia tea as a conditioner and rinsing it out after 5 minutes can help retain natural hair colour and strength.

Diabetes

Studies and researches show that Stevia may stabilize blood sugar levels, increase insulin resistance, may even promote insulin production by promoting the pancreas health, discourage glucose absorption in the blood, and inhibit candidiasis - a yeast infection that flourish with sugar. Stevia is a great low carb, low sugar and low calorie sugar alternative and the steviol glycosides are not metabolized by the body and are excreted in the urine without getting accumulated in the body. A Study also suggests that Stevia may inhibit the craving for sweet and oily or fatty foods. Drinking tea made with crushed raw Stevia leaves, or with its extract or tea bags two to three times daily may help with hyperglycemia. To make Stevia tea, heat - not boil one cup of water and let a tea bag or 1teaspoon of its leaves steep in it for 5 -7 minutes. Drink it hot or cold. Or 3-4 drops of Stevia extract can be added to warm or cold cup of water. Also stevia can be used as a natural alternative to any other artificial sweetener being used.

Gingivitis

Study shows that antibacterial properties of Stevia may help with gingivitis, cavities, tooth decay and mouth sores. It may suppress the development and reproduction of infectious organisms in the gums and teeth, inhibit the growth of plaque and may improve overall oral health. People who have used Stevia as a mouthwash has reported significant decrease in gingivitis and other mouth infections. Simply gargling with Stevia mouthwash and brushing with Stevia added toothpaste may be beneficial. To make Stevia mouthwash, add 3-4 drops of Stevia extract in half a cup of lukewarm water or steep half a cup of tea with its leaves or teabag and gargle three to four times daily especially in the morning and at night. For toothpaste, mix 2 drops of Stevia extract to the regular toothpaste.

Heartburn and Indigestion

People in Brazil, Paraguay and Bolivia have been using Stevia tea to soothe upset stomach, heartburn, and to improve indigestion and gastrointestinal function. Drinking Stevia tea after every meal may serve as a digestive aid and relieve heartburn and stomach pain.

High Blood Pressure (Hypertension)

A few longer term studies done over a period of 1 and 2 years show that stevia may lower elevated blood pressure levels. Simply drinking Stevia tea twice daily may help stabilize the blood pressure levels.

Osteoporosis

A study performed on chickens shows that by adding Stevia leaf powder to chicken feed it significantly increased calcium metabolism in the chickens and had 75% decreased eggshell breakage. A patent application for possible Osteoporosis treatment with Stevia suggests that stevia may help promote absorption of calcium in the body and help improve bone density. Suggested remedy is to make Alfalfa and stevia tea by steeping Alfalfa herb and Stevia half teaspoon each for 5-7 minutes. Drink it two to three times daily. Adding vitamin D powder to the tea or taking its supplements can be beneficial too.

Weight Loss

Recent medical research suggests that low at carbohydrates, calories and sugar Stevia may be beneficial in weight management. One preliminary research suggests that Stevia may interfere with the functions of hypothalamus and may aid weight loss by curbing the hunger sensation. Hypothalamus is a part of the brain which controls hunger, thirst and fatigue along with its other functions. Anti-glycemic activity of Stevia may also control blood glucose levels which is one of the major causes of weight gain. Stevia works as a tonic to increase energy levels in people battling for weight loss. Suggested remedy is to drink one cup of Stevia tea or mix 10-15 drops of Stevia concentrate in one cup of cold or warm water. Drink it 15 minutes before every meal.

Wrinkles and Other Skin Conditions

Stevia is believed to be a remarkable healing agent for skin disorders. Its antioxidant, antibacterial and antiseptic activity may help with wrinkles, skin blemishes, dermatitis, eczema, acne outbreaks, scarring, rashes, itchiness and chapped lips. A small amount of Stevia concentrate applied directly onto the affected skin may promote the healing process. To smooth out the wrinkles, before going to bed, apply a paste made by crushed Stevia leaves or its liquid concentrate evenly all over the face and let it dry for fifteen to twenty minutes. Wash and pat dry your face and apply a few drops of extra virgin coconut oil on the face and leave it on over night to benefit from its antioxidant effects.

What are the Side Effects of Stevia?

There are not any reported side effects of Stevia when taken in moderation. Based on intensive global researches and scientific reports, The World Health Organisation (WHO) of the UN and Food and Drug Administration of the US had approved the use of Steviol glycosides as safe and has established an acceptable daily intake of 4mg per kg of body weight. However, if you are taking any medication for diabetes or hypertension, due to its anti-glycemic and anti-hypertensive activity supervised Stevia consumption is advised. If you are pregnant or breastfeeding, consult your physician before using Stevia therapeutically.

Where and How to Buy Stevia

Stevia is available at organic grocery and herbal food stores in the form of raw dried leaves, white or green powder, sugar tabs, granulated or crystalline sugar, concentrate, and flavoured and nonflavourd liquids. When buying Stevia look for Stevia rebaudiana because it is considered the best type and the FDA approved steviol glycosides are extracted from this genus in the whole Stevia family.

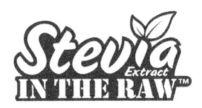

When substituting Stevia Extract In The Raw for sugar in your favorite recipes, it's important to recognize that sugar has properties other than sweetness - such as texture, moisture and browning - that may need to be compensated for when substituting Stevia Extract In The Raw.

See our cooking and baking usage tips for more information about how best to substitute Stevia Extract In The Raw for sugar in your favorite recipes.

STEVIA EXTRACT IN THE RAW™ SWEETNESS SUBSTITUTION CHART

GRANULATED SUGAR	PACKETS	CUP FOR CUP
1 TEASPOON	1/2 PACKET	1 TEASPOON
2 TEASPOONS	1 PACKET	2 TEASPOONS
1 TABLESPOON	1 1/2 PACKETS	1 TABLESPOON
1/4 CUP	6 PACKETS	1/4 CUP
1/3 CUP	8 PACKETS	1/3 CUP
1/2 CUP	12 PACKETS	1/2 CUP
2/3 CUP	16 PACKETS	2/3 CUP
3/4 CUP	18 PACKETS	3/4 CUP
1 CUP	24 PACKETS	1 CUP

Sweetness preference is a personal choice. The Substitution Chart is provided as a general guideline for using Stevia Extract In The Raw. We encourage you to experiment and develop conversion preferences based upon your palate and personal experience

www.steviaextractintheraw.com

Sugars & Substitutes with their Glycemic Index

Artificial Sweeteners	N/A	**Never a Healthy Sugar Alternative** All artificial chemical sweeteners are toxic and can indirectly lead to weight gain, the very reason many people consume them. They should be avoided. In fact, given a choice between high fructose corn syrup and artificial sweeteners, we recommend high fructose corn syrup by far (though it's essentially asking if you should consume poison or worse poison).
Yes! Stevia	0	**Best Healthy Sugar Alternative** Though it is 200-300 times sweeter than table sugar, stevia is not a sugar. Unlike other popular sweeteners, it has a glycemic index rating of less than 1 and therefore does not feed candida (yeast) or cause any of the numerous other problems associated with sugar consumption. Read more about stevia at Organic Lifestyle Magazine (OLM). Please note that Stevia and Truvia are not the same thing.
Xylito	7	Xylitol is a natural sugar alcohol sweetener found in the fibers of fruits and vegetables which can cause bloating, diarrhea, and flatulence with initial consumption. It's said to be safe for pregnant women, and is said to possibly treat ear infections, osteoposis, respiratory infections, candida, and is it even helps fight cavities. In fact, in Finland, virtually all chewing gum is sweetened with xylitol.
Agave Nectar	15-30	A sweet syrup made from the Blue Agave plant, Agave Nectar is obtained by the extraction and purification of "sap" from the agave plant, which is broken down by natural enzymes into the monosaccharides (simple sugars): mainly fructose (70-75%) and dextrose (20-26%). Read more about agave nectar at OLM.
Fructose	17	Though fructose has a low glycemic index rating, fructose consumption should be limited. Fructose is linked to heart disease as it raises triglycerides and cholesterol. It is devoid of nutrition.
Brown Rice Syrup	25	Though it is said to have a low glycemic index (25), it is not recommended for diabetics, since its sweetness comes from maltose, which is known to cause spikes in blood sugar.
Raw Honey	30	**A Healthy Sugar Alternative in moderation** With antioxidants, minerals, vitamins, amino acids, enzymes, carbohydrates, and phytonutrients, raw, unprocessed honey is considered a superfood by many alternative health care practitioners and a remedy for many health ailments. Choose your honey wisely. There is nothing beneficial about processed honey. Read more about honey at OLM.
Coconut Palm Sugar	35	Originally made from the sugary sap of the Palmyra palm, the date palm or sugar date palm (Phoenix sylvestris). It's also made from the sap of coconut palms. With a relatively low glycemic index, Cocnut palm sugar is the new rage among health nuts. It's often called "coconut nectar sugar" or "coconut sugar".

Sweetener	GI	Description
Apple Juice	40	Fresh apple juice is good for you, though we recommend eating fresh raw whole apples. Concentrated apple juice (sometimes used as a sweetener) is closer to refined sugar than fresh apple juice.
Barley Malt Syrup	42	Barley malt syrup is considered to be one of the healthiest sweeteners in the natural food industry. Barley malt is made by soaking and sprouting barley to make malt, then combining it with more barley and cooking this mixture until the starch is converted to sugar. The mash is then strained and cooked down to syrup or dried into powder.
Amasake	43	This is an ancient, Oriental whole grain sweetener made from cultured brown rice. It has a thick, pudding-like consistency. It's not easy to find in the U.S., but it is a great alternative to refined table sugar.
Sugar Cane Juice	43	Healthy Sugar Alternative in moderation. Sugar cane juice has many nutrients and other beneficial properties and is said by some health practitioners to be almost as medicinal as raw honey.
Organic Sugar	47	Organic sugar comes from sugar cane grown without the use of chemicals or pesticides. It is usually darker than traditional white sugar because it contains some molasses. (It has not been processed to the degree white sugar is processed).
Maple Syrup	54	Maple syrup is made by boiling sap collected from natural growth maple trees during March & April. It is refined sap and is therefore processed. It has a high glycemic index, and though it is much more nutritious then refined table sugar and high fructose corn syrup, there are better choices.
Evaporated Cane Juice	55	Evaporated cane juice is often considered unrefined sugar, but juicing is a refining process, and evaporating refines further. Though better than turbinado, cane juice (unevaporated) is a better choice as a sweetener.
Black Strap Molasses	55	White refined table sugar is sugar cane with all the nutrition taken out. Black strap molasses is all of that nutrition that was taken away. A quality organic (must be organic!) molasses provides iron, calcium, copper, magnesium, phosphorus, potassium and zinc, and is alkalizing to the body.
Turbinado	65	Turbinado sugar is partially processed sugar, also called raw sugar. Raw Sugar
Raw sugar	65	Raw sugar is not actually raw sugar. It is processed, though not as refined as common white table sugar. Therefore, given a choice between raw and white, choose raw. There are many different variations of raw sugar with many different names depending on how refined it is.
Cola (and most other sodas)	70	Though cola has a lower GI ranking then some might expect, there are many other reasons to avoid cola, or any type of soda. There is nothing beneficial to the human body inside a can of soda (not to mention we should avoid drinking out of aluminum cans!).
Corn Syrup	75	Corn syrup has very little nutrition and should be avoided.
Refined, Pasteurized Honey	75	The nutrition is gone, and there is often high fructose corn syrup added to processed honey. Refined pasteurized honey is no better than white table sugar.

Refined Table Sugar	80	Conventionally grown, chemically processed, and striped of all beneficial properties, many health advocates believe that refined sugar is one of the two leading causes (high fructose corn syrup is the other) of nearly every health ailment known to man (or woman or child). Not only does it have a high GI ranking, but it also is extremely acidic to the body causing calcium and other mineral depletion from bones and organs (sugar is alkaline but has a very acidic effect on the body).
High Fructose Corn Syrup	87	Many health advocates believe that high fructose corn syrup and refined sugar are the two biggest contributors to health ailments in our society. High fructose corn syrup is a combination of sucrose and fructose.
Glucose(AKA Dextrose)	100	White bread was the benchmark, but for consistency glucose now holds the rating at 100.
Maltodextrin	150	Foods that have maltodextrin often say "Low Sugar" or "Complex Carbohydrate", but this sweetener should be avoided!

Psalm 37:3, 4 says, "Trust in the Lord, and do good; so shalt thou dwell in the land, and verily thou shalt be fed.

Delight thyself also in the Lord; and he shall give thee the desires of thine heart."

Green Leafy Vegetables

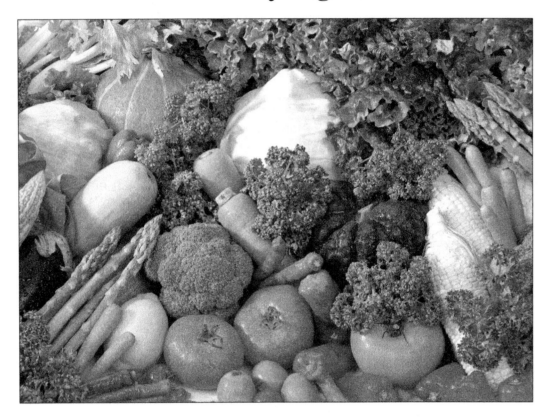

Revelation 22:2 says, "**In the midst of the street of it, and on either side of the river, was there the tree of life, which bare twelve manner of fruits, and yielded her fruit every month: and the leaves of the tree were for the healing of the nations."**

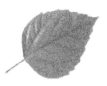

FOODS THAT PROMOTE CLEANSING

ALKALIZING VEGETABLES!

Alfalfa, Asparagus, Barley grass, Basil, Beet greens, Beets, Beetroot, Broad beans, Broccoli, Brussels Sprouts, Cabbage, Capsicum/pepper, Carrot, Cauliflower, Celery, Chard greens, Chlorella, Chili, Chives, Collard greens, Coriander, Courgette/zucchini, Cucumber, Dandelion, Dulce, Edible flowers, Eggplant/aubergine, Endive, Fermented vegetables, Garlic, Greens, Green beans, Green peas, Kale, Kelp, Kohlrabi, Lettuce, Mushrooms, Mustard greens, Nightshade Vegetables, New potatoes, Onions, Parsley, Parsnips, Peas, Peppers, Pumpkin, Radishes, Runner beans, Rutabaga, Sea vegetables, Snow peas, Spinach, Spirulina, Sprouts, String beans, Sweet potatoes, Tomatoes, Wakame, Watercress, Wheat grass and Wild greens. Alkalizing vegetables from all 7 of God's earth's continents.

Nearly one thousand species of plants with edible leaves are known. Leaf vegetables most often come from short-lived herbaceous plants such as lettuce and spinach. Woody plants whose leaves can be eaten as leaf vegetables include *Adansonia*, *Aralia*, *Moringa*, *Morus*, and *Toona* species.

ALKALIZING FRUITS!

Apple, Apricot, Avocado, Bananas, Berries, Blackberries, Cantaloupe, Cherries, Coconuts fresh, Currants, Dates, Durian, Figs, Grapes, Grapefruit, Guava, Honeydew melon, Kiwi fruit, Lemon, Lime, Mango, Muskmelons, Nectarine, Noni, Orange, Otaheite gooseberry, Papaya, Peach, Pear, Pineapple, Plums, Pomegranate, Raisins, Raspberries, Rhubarb, Strawberries, Tangerine and Watermelon. Alkalizing fruits from all 7 of God's earth's continents.

ALKALIZING PROTEIN!

Almonds, Chestnuts, Millet, Tempeh fermented, Tofu fermented, Whey Protein Powder.

ALKALIZING BREADS!

Sprouted Bread, Sprouted Wraps. Gluten & Yeast Free Breads and Wraps.

ALKALIZING SEASONINGS & SPICES!

Chili Pepper, Cinnamon, Curry, Ginger, all Herbs, Miso, Mustard, Sea Salt, Tamari and Turmeric.

ALKALIZING GRAINS & BEANS!

Amaranth, Buckwheat, Brown Rice, Chia/Salba, Kamut, Millet, Quinoa, Spelt, Lentils, Lima Beans, Mung Beans, Navy Beans, Pinto Beans, Red Beans, Soy Beans and White Beans.

ALKALIZING SPROUTS!

Alfalfa Sprouts, Amaranth Sprouts, Broccoli Sprouts, Fenugreek Sprouts, Kamut Sprouts, Mung Bean Sprouts, Quinoa Sprouts, Radish Sprouts, Soy Sprouts and Soy Sprouts.

ALKALIZING SWEETENERS

Stevia

ALKALIZING FOODS (OTHER)

Alkaline Water, Apple Cider Vinegar, Bee Pollen, Fresh Fruit Juice, Green Juices, Lecithin Granules, Mineral Water, Molasses Blackstrap, Probiotic Cultures and Vegetables Juices.

ANIMAL FLESH (MEAT) SHOULD NEVER BE MORE THAN 20% OF YOUR DAILY MEALS. ALL FLESH (MEATS) ARE ACID FOODS.

DE-SWAMP YOUR BODY. ADAPT AN 8020 DIET DAILY. 80% ALKALINE FOODS. 20% ACID FOODS.

Do not allow your taste buds to control your health. Eat with a purpose, the purpose is to feel good and stay well.

1 Corinthians 6:19 Do you not know that your body is a temple of the Holy Spirit within you, which you have from God, and that you are not your own

All of God's grapes and water melons were seeded.

Natural Organic Beans

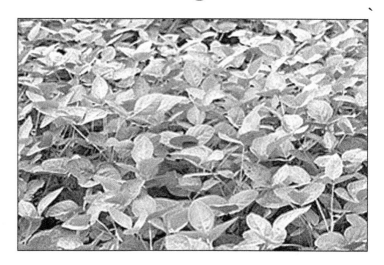

II Samuel 17:28 says, "Brought beds, and basins, and earthen vessels, and wheat, and barley, and flour, and parched corn, and beans, and lentils, and parched pulse,"

Ezekiel 4:9 says, "Take thou also unto thee wheat, and barley, and beans, and lentils, and millet, and fitches, and put them in one vessel, and make thee bread thereof, according to the number of the days that thou shalt lie upon thy side, three hundred and ninety days shalt thou eat thereof."

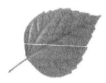

The origin of the word vegetable

"Vegetable" comes from the Latin *vegetabilis* (animated) and from *vegetare* (enliven), which is derived from *vegetus* (active), in reference to the process of a plant growing.

The word "vegetable" was first recorded in English in the 15th century,[4] and originally applied to any plant. This is still the sense of the adjective "vegetable" in biological context.[5] In 1967, the meaning of the term "vegetable" was specified to mean "plant cultivated for food, edible herb or root." The year 1955 noted the first use of the shortened, slang term "veggie". [6]

As an <u>adjective</u>, the word **vegetable** is used in scientific and technical contexts with a different and much broader meaning, namely of "related to plants" in general, edible or not — as in *vegetable matter*, *vegetable kingdom*, *vegetable origin*, etc.[5] The meaning of "vegetable" as "plant grown for food" was not established until the 18th century.[7]

Leviticus 27:27 says, "And when ye shall come into the land, and shall have planted all manner of trees for food,…"

Beautiful field of organic green leafy vegetables

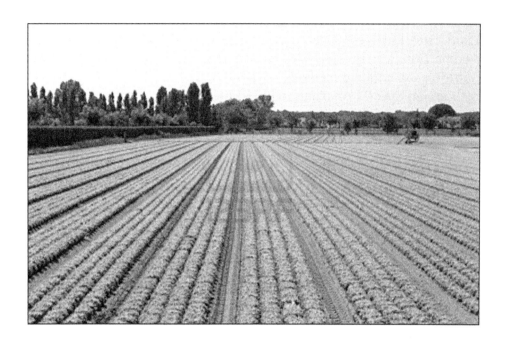

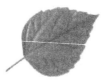

Did you know?

Leaf vegetables, also called **potherbs, green vegetables, greens,** or **leafy greens,** are plant leaves cooked and eaten as a vegetable, sometimes accompanied by tender petioles and shoots. Although they come from a very wide variety of plants, most share a great deal with other leaf vegetables in nutrition and cooking methods.

Nearly one thousand species of plants with edible leaves are known. Leaf vegetables most often come from short-lived herbaceous plants such as lettuce and spinach. Woody plants whose leaves can be eaten as leaf vegetables include *Adansonia, Aralia, Moringa, Morus,* and *Toona* species.

The leaves of many fodder crops are also edible by humans, but usually only eaten under famine conditions. Examples include alfalfa, clover, and most grasses, including wheat and barley. These plants are often much more prolific than more traditional leaf vegetables, but exploitation of their rich nutrition is difficult, primarily because of their high fiber content. This obstacle can be overcome by further processing such as drying and grinding into powder or pulping and pressing for juice.

During the first half of the 20th century, it was common for greengrocers to carry small bunches of herbs tied with a string to small green and red peppers, known as "potherbs."

Nutrition

Leaf vegetables are typically low in calories, low in fat, high in protein per calorie, high in dietary fiber, high in iron and calcium, and very high in phytochemicals such as vitamin C, carotenoids, lutein, folate as well as Vitamin K.

Preparation

Leaf vegetables may be stir-fried, stewed or steamed. Leaf vegetables stewed with chicken are a traditional dish in soul food, and southern U.S. cuisine. They are also commonly eaten in a variety of South Asian dishes such as saag. Leafy greens can be used to wrap other ingredients like a tortilla. Most leaf vegetables can also be eaten raw, for example in sandwiches or salads.[citation needed] A green smoothie enables large quantities of raw leafy greens to be consumed by blending the leaves with fruit and water.

> **Isaiah 40:6-8** the voice said, Cry. And he said, what shall I cry? All withereth, the flower fadeth: because the spirit of the Lord bloweth upon it: surely the people is grass. The grass withereth, the flower fadeth: but the word of our God shall stand for ever.flesh is grass, and all the goodliness thereof is as the flower of the field: The grass

Foods authorized by the Holy Scriptures.

Animal Protein for Meat

Calf	Proverbs 15:17; Luke 15:23
Cattle	Deuteronomy 20:14
Eggs	Job 6:6; Luke 11:12
Goat	Genesis 27:9
Lamb	2 Samuel 12:4
Oxen	1 Kings 19:21
Sheep	Deuteronomy 14:4
Venison	Genesis 27:7

Fish

John 21:6,9,10,11-13
Leviticus 11:9
Matthew 15:36

Fowl

Dove	Leviticus 12:8
Pigeon	Genesis 15:9; Leviticus 12:8
Partridge	1 Samuel 26:20; Jeremiah 17:11
Quail	Psalm 105:40

Dairy

Butter	Judges 5: 25, Proverbs 30:33
Cheese	2 Samuel 17:29; Job 10:10
Curds	Isaiah 7:15
Goat's milk	Proverbs 27:27
Milk Exodus	33:3; Job 10:10; Judges 5:25

Fruits & Nuts

Apples	Song of Solomon 2:5
Almonds	Genesis 43:11; Numbers 17:8
Dates	2 Samuel 6:19; 1 Chronicles 16:3
Figs	Nehemiah 13:15; Jeremiah 24:1-3
Grapes	Leviticus 19:10; Deuteronomy 23:24
Melons	Numbers 11:5; Isaiah 1:8
Olives	Isaiah 17:6; Micah 6:15

Fruits & Nuts Continued

Pomegranates	Numbers 20:5; Deuteronomy 8:8
Raisins	Numbers 6:3; 2 Samuel 6:19
Sycamore Fruit	Psalms 78:47; Amos 7:14

Grains

Barley	Deuteronomy 8:8; Ezekiel 4:9
Bread	Genesis 25:34; 2 Samuel 6:19; 16:1; Mark 8:14
Corn	Matthew 12:1
Flour	2 Samuel 17:28; 1 Kings 17:12
Millet	Ezekiel 4:9
Spelt	Ezekiel 4:9
Unleavened Bread	Genesis 19:3; Exodus 12:20
Wheat	Ezra 6:9; Deuteronomy 8:8

Seasoning, Spices & Herbs

Anise	Matthew 23:34
Coriander	Exodus 16:31; Number 11:7
Cinnamon	Exodus 30:23; Revelation 18:13
Cumin	Isaiah 28:25; Matthew 23:23
Dill	Matthew 23:23
Garlic	Numbers 11:5
Mint	Matthew 23:23; Luke 11:42
Mustard	Matthew 13:31
Rue	Luke 11:42
Salt	Ezra 6:9; Job 6:6

Vegetables & Legumes

Beans	2 Samuel 17:28; Ezekiel 4:9
Cucumbers	Numbers 11:5
Gourds	2 Kings 4:39
Leaf	Ezekiel 47:12
Leaves	Revelation 22:2
Leeks	Numbers 11:5
Lentils	Genesis 25:34; 2 Samuel 17:28; Ezekiel 4:9
Onions	Numbers 11:5

Other Foods

Grape Juice	Numbers 6:3
Honey	Exodus 33:3; Deuteronomy 8:8; Judges 14:8-9

Locust	Mark 1:6
Olive Oil	Ezra 6:9; Deuteronomy 8:8
Vinegar	Ruth 2:14; John 19:29
Wine	Ezra 6:9; John 2:1-10; 1 Timothy 5:23

NOTE, The word vegetable does not appear in the Holy Bible. The word vegetable does not appear anywhere prior to the 15th century. Its origin is either old French or Late Latin.

Grass Fed Beef Authorized in the Holy Bible;

- **Psalms 104:14** He causeth the grass to grow for the cattle, and herb for the service of man: that he may bring forth food out of the earth;

- **Deuteronomy 11:15** And I will send grass in thy fields for thy cattle, that thou mayest eat and be full.

Cooking oils are not mentioned or authorized in the Holy Bible.

Sugar is not mentioned or authorized in the Holy Bible.

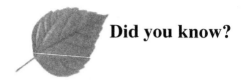 **Did you know?**

About natural weight control

Simplicity is the key to weight control. Dr. Joel Wallach states that "farmers know how to fatten things up and slim them down." If a farmer has 100 head of livestock and no plans to take that 100 head of livestock to the market. Then that farmer will be content with allowing the livestock to feed on the growing grass of the pasture. The livestock love grazing there and they stay healthy while grazing.

Deuteronomy 11:15 says "And I will send grass in thy fields for thy cattle, that thou mayest eat and be full."

Now, when the farmer's plans change relative to taking the livestock to market. He or she will now start to think in terms of maximum yield. He or she will want top dollar. They know the process well. It's been used for well over a hundred years. If you listen closely, you will hear them speak of graining them up. Meaning they bring them in from the pasture and for about 90 days they will be feeding the livestock various grains. In a few weeks the livestock will put on significant weight. Bringing top dollar at the market.

The same process works identically with humans. When humans stop eating grains, they will lose weight rather quickly and safely as well. Grains include breads, cakes, cereals, cookies, oatmeal, pies, rice, wheat and flour products as well. Dr. Joel Wallach says "A couch potato will lose weight if they eliminate all grains from their diets." However, it is vital that the individual or individuals supplement their vegetable and protein diets with Dr. Wallach's 90 essential nutrients, called the Healthy Start Kit. The 90 essential nutrients are available in Youngevity's Beyond Tangy Tangerine, Osteo-FX Plus and our E.F.A Plus Soft Gels. Item # is 10245.

To obtain Youngevity products contact Oliver Smith at 916-802-3482 or online; www.youngevityonline.com/oliversmithee

Proverbs 9:9 says, "Give instruction to a wise man, and he will be yet wiser: teach a just man, and he will increase in learning."

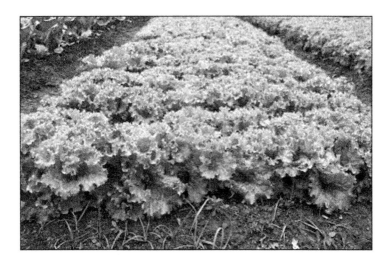

Ezekiel 47:12 says "And by the river upon the bank thereof, on this side and on that side, shall grow all trees for meat, whose leaf shall not fade, neither shall the fruit thereof be consumed: it shall bring forth new fruit according to his months, because their waters they issued out of the sanctuary: and the fruit thereof shall be for meat, **and the leaf thereof for medicine.**"

| 74TH CONGRESS | SENATE | DOCUMENT |
| 2d Session | | No. 264 |

MODERN MIRACLE MEN

AN ARTICLE

BY

REX BEACH

ENTITLED "MODERN MIRACLE MEN", RELATING TO
PROPER FOOD MINERAL BALANCES BY
DR. CHARLES NORTHEN, REPRINTED FROM
COSMOPOLITAN, JUNE 1936

PRESENTED BY MR. FLETCHER

JUNE 1 (calendar day, JUNE 5), 1936.—Ordered to be printed

UNITED STATES
GOVERNMENT PRINTING OFFICE
WASHINGTON : 1936

··· TOP SECRET ···

MODERN MIRACLE MEN

DR. CHARLES NORTHEN, WHO BUILDS HEALTH FROM THE GROUND UP

This quiet, unballyhooed pioneer and genius in the field of nutrition demonstrates that countless human ills stem from the fact that impoverished soil of America no longer provides plant foods with the mineral elements essential to human nourishment and health! To overcome this alarming condition, he doctors sick soils and, by seeming miracles, raises truly healthy and health-giving fruits and vegetables

(By Rex Beach)

Do you know that most of us today are suffering from certain dangerous diet deficiencies which cannot be remedied until the depleted soils from which our foods come are brought into *proper mineral balance?*

The alarming fact is that foods—fruits and vegetables and grains—now being raised on millions of acres of land that no longer contains enough of certain needed minerals, are starving us—no matter how much of them we eat!

This talk about minerals is novel and quite startling. In fact, a realization of the importance of minerals in food is so new that the textbooks on nutritional dietetics contain very little about it. Nevertheless, it is something that concerns all of us, and the further we delve into it the more startling it becomes.

You'd think, wouldn't you, that a carrot is a carrot—that one is about as good as another as far as nourishment is concerned? But it *isn't;* one carrot may look and taste like another and yet be lacking in the particular mineral element which our system requires and which carrots are supposed to contain. Laboratory tests prove that the fruits, the vegetables, the grains, the eggs and even the milk and the meats of today are not what they were a few generations ago. (Which doubtless explains why our forefathers thrived on a selection of foods that would starve us!) No man of today can eat enough fruits and vegetables to supply his system with the mineral salts he requires for perfect health, because his stomach isn't big enough to hold them! And we are running to big stomachs.

No longer does a balanced and fully nourishing diet consist merely of so many calories or certain vitamins or a fixed proportion of starches, proteins, and carbohydrates. We now know that *it must contain, in addition, something like a score of mineral salts.*

It is bad news to learn from our leading authorities that *99 percent of the American people are deficient in these minerals, and that a marked deficiency in any one of the more important minerals actually results in disease.* Any upset of the balance, any considerable lack of one or another element, however microscopic the body requirement may be, and we sicken, suffer, shorten our lives.

MODERN MIRACLE MEN

This discovery is one of the latest and most important contributions of science to the problem of human health.

So far as the records go, the first man in this field of research, the first to demonstrate that most human foods of our day are poor in minerals and that their proportions are not balanced, was Dr. Charles Northen, an Alabama physician now living at Orlando, Fla. His discoveries and achievements are of enormous importance to mankind.

Following a wide experience in general practice, Dr. Northen specialized in stomach diseases and nutritional disorders. Later, he moved to New York and made extensive studies along this line, in conjunction with a famous French scientist from the Sorbonne. In the course of that work he convinced himself that there was little authentic, definite information on the chemistry of foods, and that no dependence could be placed on existing data.

He asked himself how foods could be used intelligently in the treatment of disease, when they differed so widely in content. The answer seemed to be that they could not be used intelligently. In establishing the fact that serious deficiencies existed and in searching out the reasons therefor, he made an extensive study of the soil. *It was he who first voiced the surprising assertion that we must make soil building the basis of food building* in order to accomplish human building.

"Bear in mind," says Dr. Northen, "that minerals are vital to human metabolism and health—and that no plant or animal can appropriate to itself any mineral which is not present in the soil upon which it feeds.

"When I first made this statement I was ridiculed, for up to that time people had paid little attention to food deficiencies and even less to soil deficiencies. Men eminent in medicine denied there was any such thing as vegetables and fruits that did not contain sufficient minerals for human needs. Eminent agricultural authorities insisted that *all* soil contained all necessary minerals. They reasoned that plants take what they need, and that it is the function of the human body to appropriate what it requires. Failure to do so, they said, was a symptom of disorder.

"Some of our respected authorities even claimed that the so-called secondary minerals played no part whatever in human health. It is only recently that such men as Dr. McCollum of Johns Hopkins, Dr. Mendel of Yale, Dr. Sherman of Columbia, Dr. Lipman of Rutgers, and Drs. H. G. Knight and Oswald Schreiner of the United States Department of Agriculture have agreed that these minerals are essential to plant, animal, and human feeding.

"We know that vitamins are complex chemical substances which are indispensable to nutrition, and that each of them is of importance for the normal function of some special structure in the body. Disorder and disease result from any vitamin deficiency.

"It is not commonly realized, however, that vitamins control the body's appropriation of minerals, and in the absence of minerals they have no function to perform. Lacking vitamins, the system can make some use of minerals, but lacking minerals, vitamins are useless.

"Neither does the layman realize that there may be a pronounced difference in both foods and soils—to him one vegetable, one glass of milk, or one egg is about the same as another. Dirt is dirt, too, and

MODERN MIRACLE MEN

he assumes that by adding a little fertilizer to it, a satisfactory vegetable or fruit can be grown.

"The truth is that our foods vary enormously in value, and some of them aren't worth eating, as food. For example, vegetation grown in one part of the country may assay 1,100 parts, per billion, of iodine, as against 20 in that grown elsewhere. Processed milk has run anywhere from 362 parts, per million, of iodine and 127 of iron, down to nothing.

"Some of our lands, even in a virgin state, never were well balanced in mineral content, and unhappily for us, we have been systematically robbing the poor soils and the good soils alike of the very substances most necessary to health, growth, long life, and resistance to disease. Up to the time I began experimenting, almost nothing had been done to make good the theft.

"The more I studied nutritional problems and the effects of mineral deficiencies upon disease, the more plainly I saw that here lay the most direct approach to better health, and the more important it became in my mind to find a method of restoring those missing minerals to our foods.

"The subject interested me so profoundly that I retired from active medical practice and for a good many years now I have devoted myself to it. It's a fascinating subject, for it goes to the heart of human betterment."

The results obtained by Dr. Northen are outstanding. By putting back into foods the stuff that foods are made of, he has proved himself to be a real miracle man of medicine, for he has opened up the shortest and most rational route to better health.

He showed first that it should be done, and then that it could be done.

He doubled and redoubled the natural mineral content of fruits and vegetables.

He improved the quality of milk by increasing the iron and the iodine in it.

He caused hens to lay eggs richer in the vital elements.

By scientific soil feeding, he raised better seed potatoes in Maine, better grapes in California, better oranges in Florida and better field crops in other States. (By "better" is meant not only an improvement in food value but also an increase in quality and quantity.)

Before going further into the results he has obtained, let's see just what is involved in this matter of "mineral deficiencies", what it may mean to our health, and how it may affect the growth and development, both mental and physical, of our children.

We know that rats, guinea pigs, and other animals can be fed into a diseased condition and out again *by controlling only the minerals in their food.*

A 10-year test with rats proved that by withholding calcium they can be bred down to a third the size of those fed with an adequate amount of that mineral. Their intelligence, too, can be controlled by mineral feeding as readily as can their size, their bony structure, and their general health.

Place a number of these little animals inside a maze after starving some of them in a certain mineral element. The starved ones will be unable to find their way out, whereas the others will have little or no difficulty in getting out. Their dispositions can be altered by mineral

MODERN MIRACLE MEN

feeding. They can be made quarrelsome and belligerent; they can even be turned into cannibals and be made to devour each other.

A cageful of normal rats will live in amity. Restrict their calcium, and they will become irritable and draw apart from one another. Then they will begin to fight. Restore their calcium balance and they will grow more friendly; in time they will begin to sleep in a pile as before.

Many backward children are "stupid" merely because they are deficient in magnesia. We punish them for our failure to feed them properly.

Certainly our physical well-being is more directly dependent upon the minerals we take into our systems than upon calories or vitamins or upon the precise proportions of starch, protein, or carbohydrates we consume.

It is now agreed that at least *16 mineral elements are indispensable for normal nutrition*, and several more are always found in small amounts in the body, although their precise physiological role has not been determined. Of the 11 indispensable salts, calcium, phosphorus, and iron are perhaps the most important.

Calcium is the dominant nerve controller; it powerfully affects the cell formation of all living things and regulates nerve action. It governs contractility of the muscles and the rhythmic beat of the heart. It also coordinates the other mineral elements and corrects disturbances made by them. It works only in sunlight. Vitamin D is its buddy.

Dr. Sherman of Columbia asserts that *50 percent* of the American people are starving for calcium. A recent article in the Journal of the American Medical Association stated that out of 4,000 cases in New York Hospital, only 2 were not suffering from a lack of calcium.

What does such a deficiency mean? How would it affect your health or mine? So many morbid conditions and actual diseases may result that it is almost hopeless to catalog them. Included in the list are rickets, bony deformities, bad teeth, nervous disorders, reduced resistance to other diseases, fatigability, and behavior distrubances such as incorrigibility, assaultiveness, nonadaptability.

Here's one specific example: The soil around a certain Midwest city is poor in calcium. Three hundred children of this community were examined and nearly 90 percent had bad teeth, 69 percent showed affections of the nose and throat, swollen glands, enlarged or diseased tonsils, More than one-third had defective vision, round shoulders, bow legs, and anemia.

Calcium and phosphorus appear to pull in double harness. A child requires as much per day as two grown men, but studies indicate a common deficiency of both in our food. Researches on farm animals point to a deficiency of one or the other as the cause of serious losses to the farmers, and when the soil is poor in phosphorus these animals become bone-chewers. Dr. McCollum says that when there are enough phosphates in the blood there can be no dental decay.

Iron is an essential constituent of the oxygen-carrying pigment of the blood: iron starvation results in anemia, and yet iron cannot be assimilated unless some *copper* is contained in the diet. In Florida many cattle die from an obscure disease called "salt sickness." It has been found to arise from a lack of iron and copper in the soil and hence in the grass. A man may starve for want of these elements just as a beef "critter" starves.

MODERN MIRACLE MEN

If *iodine* is not present in our foods the function of the thyroid gland is disturbed and goiter afflicts us. The human body requires only fourteen-thousandths of a milligram daily, yet we have a distinct "goiter belt" in the Great Lakes section, and in parts of the Northwest the soil is so poor in iodine that the disease is common.

So it goes, down through the list, each mineral element playing a definite role in nutrition. A characteristic set of symptoms, just as specific as any vitamin-deficiency disease, follows a deficiency in any one of them. It is alarming, therefore, to face the fact that we are starving for these precious, health-giving substances.

Very well, you say, if our foods are poor in the mineral salts they are supposed to contain, why not resort to dosing?

That is precisely what is being done, or being attempted. However, those who should know assert that the human system cannot appropriate those elements to the best advantage in any but the food form. At best, only a part of them in the form of drugs can be utilized by the body, and certain dietitians go so far as to say it is a waste of effort to fool with them. Calcium, for instance, cannot be supplied in any form of medication with lasting effect.

But there is a more potent reason why the curing of diet deficiencies by drugging hasn't worked out so well. Consider those 16 indispensable elements and those others which presumably perform some obscure function as yet undetermined. Aside from calcium and phosphorus, they are needed only in infinitesimal quantities, and the activity of one may be dependent upon the presence of another. To determine the precise requirements of each individual case and to attempt to weigh it out on a druggist's scales would appear hopeless.

It is a problem and a serious one. But here is the hopeful side of the picture: *Nature can and will solve it if she is encouraged to do so.* The minerals in fruit and vegetables are colloidal; i. e., they are in a state of such extremely fine suspension that they can be assimilated by the human system: It is merely a question of giving back to nature the materials with which she works.

We must rebuild our soils: Put back the minerals we have taken out. That sounds difficult but it isn't. Neither is it expensive. Therein lies the short cut to better health and longer life.

When Dr. Northen first asserted that many foods were lacking in mineral content and that this deficiency was due solely to an absence of those elements in the soil, his findings were challenged and he was called a crank. But differences of opinion in the medical profession are not uncommon—it was only 60 years ago that the Medical Society of Boston passed a resolution condemning the use of bathtubs—and he persisted in his assertion that inasmuch as foods did not contain what they were supposed to contain, no physician could with certainty prescribe a diet to overcome physical ills.

He showed that the textbooks are not dependable because many of the analyses in them were made many years ago, perhaps from products raised in virgin soils, whereas our soils have been constantly depleted. Soil analyses, he pointed out, reflect only the content of samples. One analysis may be entirely different from another made 10 miles away.

"And so what?" came the query.

Dr. Northen undertook to demonstrate that something could be done about it. *By reestablishing a proper soil balance he actually grew crops that contained an ample amount of the desired minerals.*

MODERN MIRACLE MEN

This was incredible. It was contrary to the books and it upset everything connected with diet practice. The scoffers began to pay attention to him. Recently the Southern Medical Association, realizing the hopelessness of trying to remedy nutritional deficiencies without positive factors to work with, recommended a careful study to determine the real mineral content of foodstuffs and the variations due to soil depletion in different localities. These progressive medical men are awake to the importance of prevention.

Dr. Northen went even further and proved that crops grown in a properly mineralized soil were bigger and better; that seeds germinated quicker, grew more rapidly and made larger plants; that trees were healthier and put on more fruit of better quality.

By increasing the mineral content of citrus fruit he likewise improved its texture, its appearance and its flavor.

He experimented with a variety of growing things, and in every case the story was the same. By mineralizing the feed at poultry farms, he got more and better eggs; by balancing pasture soils, he produced richer milk. Persistently he hammered home to farmers, to doctors, and to the general public the thought that life depends upon the minerals.

His work led him into a careful study of the effects of climate, sunlight, ultraviolet and thermal rays upon plant, animal, and human hygiene. In consequence he moved to Florida. People familiar with his work consider him the most valuable man in the State. I met him by reason of the fact that I was harassed by certain soil problems on my Florida farm which had baffled the best chemists and fertilizer experts available.

He is an elderly, retiring man, with a warm smile and an engaging personality. He is a trifle shy until he opens up on his pet topic; then his diffidence disappears and he speaks with authority. His mind is a storehouse crammed with precise, scientific data about soil and food chemistry, the complicated life processes of plants, animals, and human beings—and the effect of malnutrition upon all three. He is perhaps as close to the secret of life as any man anywhere.

"Do you call yourself a soil or a food chemist?" I inquired.

"Neither. I'm an M. D. My work lies in the field of biochemistry and nutrition. I gave up medicine because this is a wider and a more important work. Sick soils mean sick plants, sick animals, and sick people. Physical, mental, and moral fitness depends largely upon an ample supply and a proper proportion of the minerals in our foods. Nerve function, nerve stability, nerve cell-building likewise depend thereon. I'm really a doctor of sick soils."

"Do you mean to imply that the vegetables I'm raising on my farm are sick?" I asked.

"Precisely! They're as weak and undernourished as anemic children. They're not much good as food. Look at the pests and the diseases that plague them. Insecticides cost farmers nearly as much as fertilizer these days.

"A healthy plant, however, grown in soil properly balanced, *can and will resist most insect pests*. That very characteristic makes it a better food product. You have tuberculosis and pneumonia germs in your system but you're strong enough to throw them off. Similarly, a really healthy plant will pretty nearly take care of itself in

MODERN MIRACLE MEN

the battle against insects and blights—and will also give the human system what it requires."

"Good heavens! Do you realize what that means to agriculture?"

"Perfectly. Enormous savings. Better crops. Lowered living costs to the rest of us. But I'm not so much interested in agriculture as in health."

"It sounds beautifully theoretical and utterly impractical to me," I told the doctor, whereupon he gave me some of his case records.

For instance, in an orange grove infested with scale, when he restored the mineral balance to part of the soil, the trees growing in that part became clean while the rest remained diseased. By the same means he had grown healthy rosebushes between rows that were riddled by insects.

He had grown tomato and cucumber plants, both healthy and diseased, where the vines intertwined. The bugs ate up the diseased and refused to touch the healthy plants! He showed me interesting analyses of citrus fruit, the chemistry and the food value of which accurately reflected the soil treatment the trees had received.

There is no space here to go fully into Dr. Northen's work but it is of such importance as to rank with that of Burbank, the plant wizard, and with that of our famous physiologists and nutritional experts.

"Healthy plants mean healthy people", said he. "We can't raise a strong race on a weak soil. Why don't you try mending the deficiencies on your farm and growing more minerals into your crops?"

I did try and I succeeded. I was planting a large acreage of celery and under Dr. Northen's direction I fed minerals into certain blocks of the land in varying amounts. When the plants from this soil were mature I had them analyzed, along with celery from other parts of the State. It was the most careful and comprehensive study of the kind ever made, and it included over 250 separate chemical determinations. I was amazed to learn that my celery had more than twice the mineral content of the best grown elsewhere. Furthermore, it kept much better, with and without refrigeration, proving that the cell structure was sounder.

In 1927, Mr. W. W. Kincaid, a "gentleman farmer" of Niagara Falls, heard an address by Dr. Northen and was so impressed that he began extensive experiments in the mineral feeding of plants and animals. The results he has accomplished are conspicuous. He set himself the task of increasing the iodine in the milk from his dairy herd. He has succeeded in adding both iodine and iron so liberally that one glass of his milk contains all of these minerals that an adult man requires for a day.

Is this significant? Listen to these incredible figures taken from a bulletin of the South Carolina Food Research Commission: "In many sections *three out of five persons* have goiter and a recent estimate states that *30 million people in the United States suffer from it.*"

Foods rich in iodine are of the greatest importance to these sufferers.

Mr. Kincaid took a brown Swiss heifer calf which was dropped in the stockyards, and by raising her on mineralized pasturage and a properly balanced diet made her the third all-time champion of her breed! In one season she gave 21,924 pounds of milk. He raised

MODERN MIRACLE MEN

her butterfat production from 410 pounds in 1 year to 1,037 pounds. Results like these are of incalculable importance.

Others besides Mr. Kincaid are following the trail Dr. Northen blazed. Similar experiments with milk have been made in Illinois and nearly every fertilizer company is beginning to urge use of the rare mineral elements. As an example I quote from statements of a subsidiary of one of the leading copper companies:

> Many States show a marked reduction in the productive capacity of the soil * * * in many districts amounting to a 25 to 50 percent reduction in the last 50 years * * *. Some areas show a tenfold variation in calcium. Some show a sixtyfold variation in phosphorus * * *. Authorities * * * see soil depletion, barren livestock, increased human death rate due to heart disease, deformities, arthritis, increased dental caries, all due to lack of essential minerals in plant foods.

"It is neither a complicated nor an expensive undertaking to restore our soils to balance and thereby work a real miracle in the control of disease," says Dr. Northen. "As a matter of fact, it's a money-making move for the farmer, and any competent soil chemist can tell him how to proceed.

"First determine by analysis the precise chemistry of any given soil, then correct the deficiencies by putting down enough of the missing elements to restore its balance. The same care should be used as in prescribing for a sick patient, for *proportions are of vital importance.*

"In my early experiments I found it extremely difficult to get the variety of minerals needed in the form in which I wanted to use them but advancement in chemistry, and expecially our ever-increasing knowledge of colloidal chemistry, has solved that difficulty. It is now possible, by the use of minerals in colloidal form, to prescribe a cheap and effective system of soil correction which meets this vital need and one which fits in admirably with nature's plans.

"Soils seriously deficient in minerals cannot produce plant life competent to maintain our needs, and with the continuous cropping and shipping away of those concentrates, the condition becomes worse.

"A famous nutrition authority recently said, 'One sure way to end the American people's susceptibility to infection is to supply through food a balanced ration or iron, copper, and other metals. An organism supplied with a diet adequate to, or preferably in excess of, all mineral requirements may so utilize these elements as to produce immunity from infection quite beyond anything we are able to produce artificially by our present method of immunization. You can't make up the deficiency by using patent medicine.'

"He's absolutely right. Prevention of disease is easier, more practical, and more economical than cure, but not until foods are standardized on a basis of what they contain instead of what they look like can the dietitian prescribe them with intelligence and with effect.

"There was a time when medical therapy had no standards because the therapeutic elements in drugs had not been definitely determined on a chemical basis. Pharmaceutical houses have changed all that. Food chemistry, on the other hand, has depended almost entirely upon governmental agencies for its research, and in our real knowledge of values we are about where medicine was a century ago.

"Disease preys most surely and most viciously on the undernourished and unfit plants, animals, and human beings alike, and when the importance of these obscure mineral elements is fully realized the

MODERN MIRACLE MEN

chemistry of life will have to be rewritten. No man knows his mental or bodily capacity, how well he can feel or how long he can live, for we are all cripples and weaklings. It is a disgrace to science. Happily, that chemistry is being rewritten and we're on our way to better health by returning to the soil the things we have stolen from it.

"*The public can help; it can hasten the change.* How? By demanding quality in its food. By insisting that our doctors and our health departments establish scientific standards of nutritional value.

"The growers will quickly respond. They can put back those minerals almost overnight, and by doing so they can actually make money through bigger and better crops.

"It is simpler to cure sick soils than sick people—which shall we choose?"

○

Introduction to a Collection of Healthy Recipes

The following recipes consist of ingredients known to be free of irritants, toxins and carcinogens, when said ingredients are acquired from a reliable natural organic source.

Among all of the ingredients in the reciples, you will NOT find, carbonated drinks, margarine, artificial butters, processed sugars or sugar substitutes, glutens, fried foods or any heated oils, burnt or over cooked meats, any lunch meats containing sodium nitrates or nitrites, artificial meats or any GMO's Genetically Modified Organisms or GMI's Genetically Modified Ingredients.

Readers are encouraged to adjust portions as needed. Creativity is encouraged when using the recipes from this book providing the preparation parameters are respected.

BREAKFAST

Ezekiel Blueberry Pancakes
French toast Ezekiel Bread
Grapefruit & Eggs
Heaven's Breakfast
Eggs Sunnyside Up with Ezekiel Toast
Divine Breakfast
Breakfast from God's Garden

ENTREES

CCC Salmon Salad
Broiled Beef Steak
Garlic Chicken
Broiled Salmon Fillets
Sea Bass Broiled With Salad
Broiled Lamb Chops
Daniel's Salad
Cheese Burger on Ezekiel
Hamburger on Ezekiel Bun

EZEKIEL BLUEBERRY PANCAKES

Ingredients

2 cups of Handy Pantry Sprouting Organic Ezekiel bread making mix*
2 cups of milk
2 to 3 free range chicken eggs
2 teaspoons baking powder
1 teaspoon of sea salt
¼ to ½ cup of olive oil, butter
1 cup of fresh blueberries

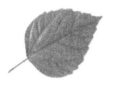
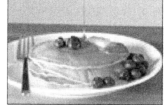

Preparations
Mix and beat ingredients together, cook as usual on low heat.
Prepare green salad to be served with Ezekiel pancakes.

*Basic Ezekiel Bread Making Kit

- 5 lbs Ezekiel Grain Mix
- 1.5 lbs Ezekiel Sprout Mix
- 1 Quart Sprouting Jar
- Laminated Ezekiel Bread Recipe Card

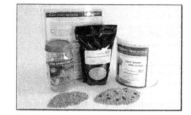

http://www.wheatgrasskits.com/ezekiel_bread_making_kits.htm

Natural Syrups Sweetened With Stevia

Stevia Blueberry Syrup

Stevia Blackberry Syrup

Stevia Cherry Syrup

Stevia Grape Syrup

Stevia Maple Syrup Maple Syrup

Stevia Strawberry Syrup

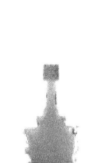

http://www.naturesflavors.com/default.php?cPath=231 1-714-744-3700

Home juicing brings great natural value to our health. Drinking water is essential for good health as well.

OPTIONAL / Sliced apple, Sliced orange or Sliced cantaloupe.

FRENCH TOAST EZEKIEL BREAD

Ingredients

8 slices of Ezekiel Bread
2 to 3 free range chicken eggs
Ground cinnamon seasoning
¼ lb. stick of butter
½ cup of milk
1 teaspoon of Stevia

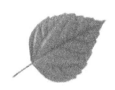
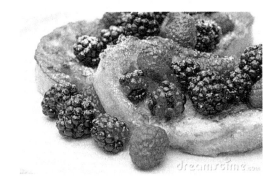

Preparations

Beat eggs, milk, and cinnamon together in a 10 inch bowl. Heat a 12 to 16 inch stainless steel or cast iron skillet low temperature. Dip each slice of bread into the egg mixture, allowing the bread to soak up some of the mixture. Adjust heat between low to medium as needed to brown French bread. Melt 3 to 4 1/8 inch thick pads of butter in the heated skillet. Cook until brown on both sides, flipping the bread when necessary.

Prepare a green salad to be served with the French toast.

Serve hot with butter and with any 1 of Stevia's berry syrups.

Home juicing brings great natural nutritional value to our health. Carrots, apples and vegetables are great for juicing. Drinking water is essential for good health as well.

OPTIONAL / Sliced apple, Strawberries or Sliced watermelon.

Natural Syrups Sweetened With Stevia

Stevia Blueberry Syrup

Stevia Blackberry Syrup

Stevia Cherry Syrup

Stevia Grape Syrup

Stevia Lemon Syrup

Stevia Strawberry Syrup   Stevia Mample Syrup

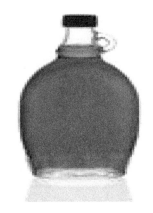

Source of Stevia; Trader Joe's, Nature's Flavors.com 1-714-744-3700
http://www.naturesflavors.com/default.php?cPath=231

GRAPEFRUIT & EGGS

Ingredients

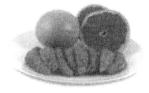

6 free range chicken eggs
1 medium to large grapefruit cut in half
Powdered Stevia
4 slices of Ezekiel Bread
¼ lb stick of butter.

Preparations

Boil 1 quart of water. Insert the six eggs into the boiling water. Boil eggs for 3 to 4 minutes or as desired. Toast Ezekiel Bread while eggs are boiling.

Serve eggs and season with Bragg Organic Sprinkle or sea salt. Add toasted bread to the plate. Sprinkle powdered Stevia to the grapefruit halves.
Make fresh grapefruit juice at home for freshness

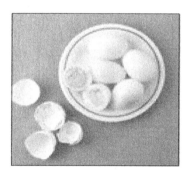

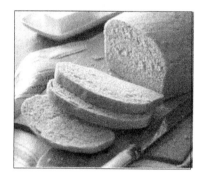

HEAVEN'S BREAKFAST

Ingredients

½ cup of chopped broccoli
¼ cup chopped onion & 4 cloves of garlic, minced
½ cup grated carrots
¼ cup chopped celery
¼ cup chopped green bell pepper
1-tablespoon parsley leaves, fresh chopped
1 medium chopped tomatoe
Sliced tomatoes
4 leafs of lettuce
½ to 1 pound of grass fed ground beef

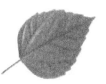
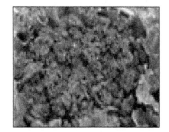

Preparations

Heat a stainless steel or cast iron skillet over low heat. Place ground beef into the heated skillet. Use a stainless steel spatulas stirring continuously not allowing the beef to stick to the bottom of the skillet. As the beef browns slightly, pour the chopped ingredients over the browning ground beef. Continue to stir not allowing any sticking or over cooking. It is essential for vegetables to maintain their crispness. Serve sliced tomatoes and lettuce.

Home juicing brings great natural value to our health. Drinking water is essential for good health as well.

OPTIONAL: Sliced kiwi fruit, Sliced orange or sliced honeydew melon. Serve sprouted bread or Ezekiel Bread.

Bragg Liquid Aminos / Natural Soy Sauce Alternative / Gluten – Free
Contains No Preservatives / Certified NON-GMO.

Bragg Organic Sprinkle / 24 Herbs & Spices Seasoning

Bragg Organic Apple Cider Vinegar

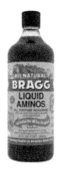
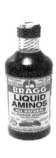
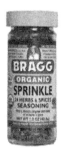
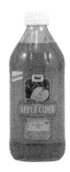

EGGS SUNNYSIDE UP WITH EZEKIEL TOAST

Ingredients

4 to 6 free range chicken eggs
4 to 8 slices of Ezekiel Bread
1 to 2 sticks of ¼ lb sticks of butter
2 tomatoes
Romaine lettuce
2 medium carrots
2 stalks of celery
1 beet

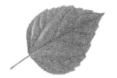
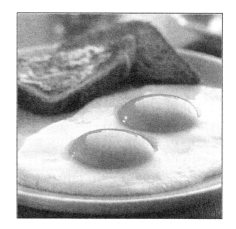

Preparations

For major nutrients and balance serve a salad with the eggs and toast. Chop 2 tomatoes, Chop romaine lettuce. Grate 2 carrots. Chop 2 stalks of celery. Peel and chop beet. Mix salad ingredients in a large salad bowl.

Heat a stainless steel or cast iron skillet over low heat. Melt 8 1/8 inch thick pads of butter in the heated skillet. Break eggs into heated melted butter, low heat. Cover skillet with lid. Every 30 to 45 seconds ease stainless steel spatulas between the skillet and the bottom of the eggs to prevent the eggs from sticking to the skillet and without breaking the yolks. Replace the lid onto the skillet for 30 to 45 seconds. Toast Ezekiel Bread in the broiler to desired brownness, with butter. Check eggs with spatulas to prevent sticking and replace lid to skillet. When eggs yolks have reached the desired softness or firmness without over cooking, remove eggs to serving plate. Season eggs to taste with Bragg Organic Sprinkle. Use Bragg Ginger & Sesame salad dressing.

Serve eggs and toast hot with salad and enjoy a very healthy breakfast

OPTIONAL / Serve figs or nectarines

Bragg Organic Sprinkle / 24 Herbs & Spices Seasoning

Salad dressing, Bragg Made with Organic, Ginger & Sesame

Orange juice made at home assures freshness when you start with fresh orange

DIVINE BREAKFAST

Ingredients

½ cup of chopped cauliflower
¼ cup of turmeric, minced
Sliced red bell pepper
¼ cup of garlic, minced
½ cup of chopped leeks
¼ cup of chopped celery
½ cup of chopped tomatoes
¼ cup of grated carrots
¼ - ½ teaspoon chili powder
2 tablespoon Bragg Organic Apple Cider Vinegar
4 to 6 poached free-range chicken eggs

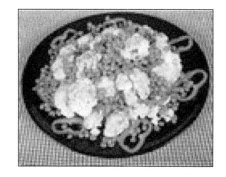

Preparations

Heat a stainless steel or cast iron skillet over low heat. Place 1/16 of a cup of water into the heated skillet along with 2 tablespoons of butter. Allow butter to melt. Place chopped vegetables into the skillet. Stirring with stainless steel spatulas. Add Bragg Organic Apple Cider Vinegar to vegetables. Do not over cook. It is essential that the vegetables retain their crispness.

While vegetables are cooking, heat another pan that is at least 3-inches so there is enough water to cover the eggs. Also make sure the pan is wide enough for the eggs you are poaching. Break the eggs into a bowl. Bring the water to a boil. Then reduce the heat to a simmer. Slowly pour the eggs from the bowl into the hot water without breaking the yolks. Using a slotted spoon or spatulas spinning the water while keeping the egg whites together and to keep the eggs from sticking to the bottom of the pan as well. Eggs should cook from 2 to 4 minutes or as desired.

Place cooked vegetables and poached eggs onto a serving plate. Season eggs with Bragg Organic Sprinkle to taste.

Home juicing brings great natural value to our health. Drinking water is essential for good health as well.

OPTIONAL / Serve sliced pears or grapes. Serve toasted Ezekiel bread with butter if desired.
Bragg Liquid Aminos / Natural Soy Sauce Alternative / Gluten – Free
Contains No Preservatives / Certified NON-GMO.

Bragg Organic Sprinkle / 24 Herbs & Spices Seasoning

BREAKFAST FROM GOD'S GARDEN

Ingredients

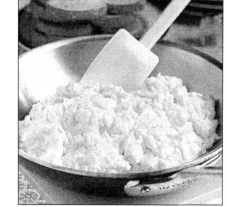

¼ **of a medium head of green or red cabbage chopped**
¼ cup chopped onion & 3 cloves of garlic
¼ cup of chopped green, red or yellow bell pepper
¼ cup of grated sharp cheddar cheese
1/8 teaspoon of sea salt
4 to 6 free range chicken eggs
Blueberries and strawberries
Sliced avocado
Sliced tomatoes

Preparations

4 to 6 free range chicken eggs, scramble in a 2 qt stainless steel or glass bowl. Chop ¼ of medium head of green or red cabbage. ¼ cup chopped onion, 3 cloves of garlic chopped. Chopped ¼ cup of green, red or yellow bell peppers, ¼ cup of grated sharp cheddar cheese, 1/8 teaspoon of sea salt.
Cover the bottom of a 10" stainless steel or cast iron skillet with 1/8 inch of water. Heat water to the point of steam and a low boil. Pour scrambled or beaten eggs into heated skillet. Reduce heat under skillet. Using stainless steel spatulas, stirring continuously not allowing the eggs to stick to the bottom of the skillet.
After cooking the eggs for about 60 to 90 seconds pour all of the chopped ingredients into the skillet with the eggs. Continue to stir not allowing any sticking to the skillet. When the eggs are cooked to a soft scramble, pour ingredients of the skillet on a serving plate. Serve with sliced tomatoes, sliced avocado, blueberries and strawberries.

Home juicing brings great natural value to our health. Drinking water is essential for good health as well.

OPTIONAL / Sliced apple, sliced orange or sliced cantaloupe. Serve sprouted bread or Ezekiel Bread.

Bragg Liquid Aminos / Natural Soy Sauce Alternative / Gluten – Free
Contains No Preservatives / Certified NON-GMO.
Bragg Organic Sprinkle / 24 Herbs & Spices Seasoning
Bragg Organic Apple Cider Vinegar

Cooking with butter at low temperature is also a healthy option when scrambling eggs.

ENTREES CCC SALMON SALAD

Ingredients

1 pound of fresh salmon, cooked in the over for 15 minutes and let cool
¼ cup fresh organic yellow corn
3 tablespoons of Bragg Organic Aminos
2 tablespoons of lime juice
2 tablespoons of olive oil
2 packets of Stevia
8 cups loosely packed mesclun salad greens
1 cup thinly sliced carrot
1 cup thinly sliced avocado
¼ cup loosely packed cilantro leaves

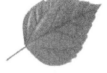

Preparations

Mix the Bragg Organic Aminos, limejuice, olive oil and Stevia until well blended. Set aside for a moment.

Place the salad greens in a large platter. Separate the salmon in thin slices. Add salmon to the platter along with the avocado, carrot, cilantro leaves and corn. Toss gently with enough dressing to coat the ingredients. Add more dressing to taste.

Home juicing brings great natural value to our health. Drinking water is essential for good health as well.

Ezekiel Bread and butter.

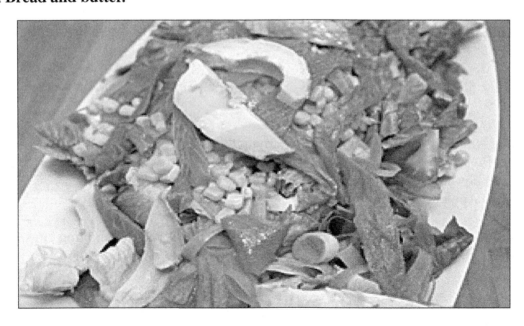

ENTREES BROILED BEEF STEAK

Ingredients

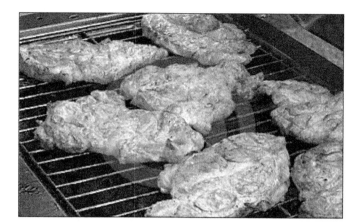

2 - 4 grass fed beef steaks, 8 oz.
2 elongated heads of Romaine lettuce
3 cloves of garlic, chopped
2 tomatoes, sliced and chopped
2 medium carrots, grated
2 stalks of celery, chopped
1 cucumber, sliced thin
1 medium leek, peel and use white portion only, thinly sliced
¼ cup of grated sharp cheddar cheese
3 lemons
Bragg Liquid Aminos
Salad dressing, Bragg Made with Organic, Ginger & Sesame

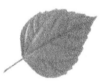

Preparations

Prepare ingredients and make salad in a large salad bowl. Store salad in the refrigerator until the steaks are ready to serve.

Broil 8 oz steaks in the oven broiler or on a grill, until steaks are cooked as desired. Season to taste with Bragg Organic Sprinkle. Do not over cook.

Lemonade - Cut lemons into halves. Squeeze lemon juice into a 2 or 3-quart pitcher. Remove the seeds from the pitcher. Fill the pitcher with water. Sweeten the lemon water with Stevia to the desired level of sweetness

OPTIONAL / Bragg Healthy Vinaigrette. 2. Bragg Organic Hawaiian, Fat Free Dressing & Marinade. 3. Bragg Organic BraggBerry.

Ezekiel Bread and butter

http://bragg.com/products/bragg-organic-hawaiian-salad-dressing.html

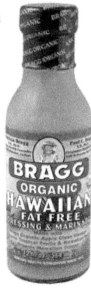

ENTREES GARLIC CHICKEN

Ingredients

¼ cup of minced garlic
½ cup of chopped celery
¼ cup of chopped green peppers
1 chopped tomatoes
1-teaspoon ground cumin
½ a head of shredded cabbage
4 free range chicken breasts with skin
1/8 teaspoon of sea salt
3 lemons

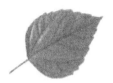
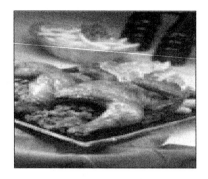

Preparations

1. Mix minced garlic, chopped celery, chopped green peppers, chopped tomatoes, and cumin, sea salt and ¼ cup of Bragg Liquid Aminos in a bowl.

2. Place the 4 chicken breasts in a stainless steel or cast iron skillet. Pour ¼ of an inch of water into the skillet. Lightly season the chicken breast with Bragg Organic Sprinkle.

3. Place the covered skillet into an oven pre-heated to 325°F for about 25 minutes. Remove skillet from oven and pour the ingredients of the bowl over the chicken breast. Place the skillet back into the oven for another 20 minutes. Remove skillet from oven.

4. Spread shredded cabbage over serving platter. Pour the contents of the skillet over the shredded cabbage.

Cut lemons into halves. Squeeze lemon juice into a 2 or 3-quart pitcher. Remove the seeds from the pitcher. Fill the pitcher with water. Sweeten the lemon water with Stevia to the desired level of sweetness.

Serve buttered Ezekiel Bread.

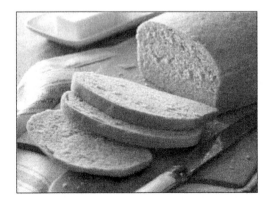

ENTREES BROILED SALMON FILLETS

Ingredients

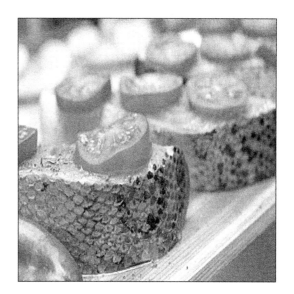

2 – 2lbs salmon fillets
2 elongated heads of Romaine lettuce
2 tomatoes, sliced and chopped
2 medium carrots, grated
2 stalks of celery, chopped
1 cucumber, sliced thin
¼ cup sliced radish
1 medium leek, peel and use white-
Portion only, thinly
¼ cup of grated sharp cheddar cheese
3 lemons
Bragg Liquid Aminos
Salad dressing, Bragg Healthy Vinaigrette

Preparations

Prepare ingredients and make salad in a large salad bowl. Store salad in the refrigerator until the fillets are ready to serve.

Broil salmon fillets in the oven broiler or on a grill, until salmon fillets are cooked as desired. Season fillets with Bragg Organic Sprinkle. Do not over cook.

Cut 3 lemons into halves. Squeeze lemon juice into a 2 or 3-quart pitcher. Remove the seeds from the pitcher. Fill the pitcher with water. Sweeten the lemon water with Stevia to the desired level of sweetness.

OPTIONAL, Serve sliced apple and or pears.
Ezekiel Bread and butter

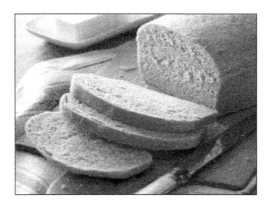

ENTREES: SEABASS BROILED WITH SALAD

Ingredients

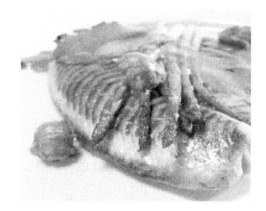

2 pounds sea bass
¼ tablespoon of garlic powder
¼ tablespoon of onion powder
1/8 teaspoon of cayenne pepper
3 large cloves garlic, chopped
5 to 10 of asparagus spears
4-tablespoon butter
¼ teaspoon sea salt
2 tablespoon of extra virgin olive oil
¼ tablespoon Bragg Organic Sprinkle

Preparations

Preheat oven or grill. In a bowl, stir together Bragg Sprinkle, garlic powder, onion powder, cayenne pepper and sea salt. Sprinkle seasoning over entire fish. Steam asparagus for 4 to 5 minutes.
In a saucepan, melt the butter with the garlic. When butter has melted remove from heat. Lightly oil the surface of the pan or the grill grate. Cook fish for about 6 minutes while drizzling with butter on both sides of the fish. Cover fish with asparagus. Use all of the oil before serving.

Ingredients

2 elongated heads of Romaine lettuce
2 tomatoes, sliced and chopped
2 medium carrots, grated
2 stalks of celery, chopped
1 cucumber, sliced thin
¼ cup sliced radish
1 medium leek, peel and use white portion only, thinly
¼ cup of grated sharp cheddar cheese
3 lemons
Salad dressing, Bragg Healthy Vinaigrette
Prepare ingredients and make salad in a large salad bowl. Store salad in the refrigerator until the fillets are ready to serve.
Cut 3 lemons into halves. Squeeze lemon juice into a 2 or 3-quart pitcher. Remove the seeds from the pitcher. Fill the pitcher with water. Sweeten the lemon water with Stevia to the desired level of sweetness.
Ezekiel Bread and butter

ENTREES **BROILED LAMB CHOPS**

Ingredients

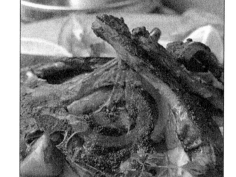

4 to 6 lamb chops
2 elongated heads of Romaine lettuce
3 cloves of garlic, chopped
2 tomatoes, sliced and chopped
2 medium carrots, grated
2 stalks of celery, chopped
1 cucumber, sliced thin
1 medium leek, peel and use white portion only, thinly
¼ cup of grated sharp cheddar cheese
3 lemons
Bragg Liquid Aminos
Salad dressing, Bragg Made with Organic, Ginger & Sesame
Reese's Mint Sauce

Preparations

Prepare ingredients and make salad in a large salad bowl. Store salad in the refrigerator until the chops are ready to serve.

Marinade lamb shops in Reese's Mint Sauce for 20 minutes. Broil lamb chops in the oven broiler or on a grill, until chops are cooked as desired. Season lightly, with Bragg Organic Sprinkle. Do not over cook.

Lemonade - Cut lemons into halves. Squeeze lemon juice into a 2 or 3-quart pitcher. Remove the seeds from the pitcher. Fill the pitcher with water. Sweeten the lemon water with Stevia to the desired level of sweetness

OPTIONAL / Serve sliced cantaloupe
Ezekiel Bread and butter

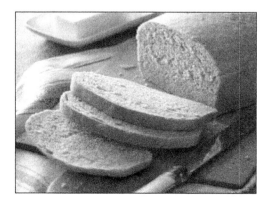

ENTREES DANIEL'S SALAD

Ingredients

1 head lettuce chopped
1 beets, peeled and chopped
1 scallion, chopped
2 stalks celery, chopped
¼ bunch of spinach, chopped
½ parsley, chopped
½ cups mushrooms, chopped
¼ cucumbers, sliced and chopped
2 cloves of garlic, chopped
½ cup of sprouts, chopped
3 tomatoes, sliced and chopped
Quartered boiled eggs from free-range chickens

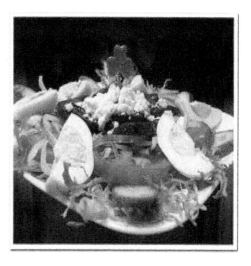

Preparations

Place ingredients into a large salad bowl; mix Bragg Organic Hawaiian salad dressing into ingredients well. The Daniel's Salad is ready to be served.

Lemonade - Cut lemons into halves. Squeeze lemon juice into a 2 or 3-quart pitcher. Remove the seeds from the pitcher. Fill the pitcher with water. Sweeten the lemon water with Stevia to the desired level of sweetness

Bragg Organic Sprinkle / 24 Herbs & Spices Seasoning

OPTIONAL Bragg Organic Hawaiian salad dressing

Serve with sliced watermelon and bananas

Ezekiel Bread and butter /

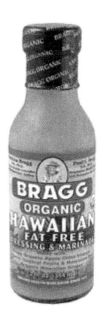

CHEESE BURGER ON EZEKIEL BUN

Ingredients

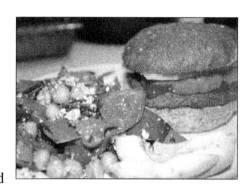

1 pound of grass fed ground beef
3 whole tomatoes, 1 sliced and 2 chopped
2 heads of Romaine lettuce
1 sliced avocados
2 carrots, grated
2 stalks of celery, chopped
1 cucumber, thinly sliced
1 medium leek, peel and use white portion only, thinly sliced
1 pound block natural of cheddar cheese
¼ cup of sharp cheddar cheese
¼ cup of garbanzo beans
3 lemons
Bragg Liquid Aminos
Salad dressing, Bragg Made with Organic, Ginger & Sesame
Ezekiel Buns

Preparations

Prepare ingredients and make salad in a large salad bowl. Store salad in the refrigerator until the hamburgers are ready to serve. Slice cheese for hamburgers.

Broil hamburger patty in the oven broiler or on a grill, until hamburger are cooked as desired. Season to taste with Bragg Organic Sprinkle and Bragg Liquid Aminos. Place cheese on hamburger. Do not over cook. Place hamburgers on Ezekiel buns, place sliced tomatoes on hamburgers, followed by 2 to 4 leafs of Romaine lettuce to size of burger. Use a natural mustard or mayonnaise and serve.

Lemonade - Cut lemons into halves. Squeeze lemon juice into a 2 or 3-quart pitcher. Remove the seeds from the pitcher. Fill the pitcher with water. Sweeten the lemon water with Stevia to the desired level of sweetness

OPTIONAL; Bragg Healthy Vinaigrette. 2. Bragg Organic Hawaiian, Fat Free Dressing & Marinade. 3. Bragg Organic BraggBerry.

Ezekiel Bread and butter

http://bragg.com/products/bragg-organic-hawaiian-salad-dressing.html

HAMBURGER ON EZEKIEL BUN

Ingredients

1 pound of grass fed ground beef
3 whole tomatoes, 1 sliced and 2 chopped
2 heads of Romaine lettuce
2 carrots, grated
2 stalks of celery, chopped
1 cucumber, thinly sliced
1 thinly sliced onion
¼ cup of sharp cheddar cheese
3 lemons
Bragg Liquid Aminos
Salad dressing, Bragg Made with Organic, Ginger & Sesame
Ezekiel Buns

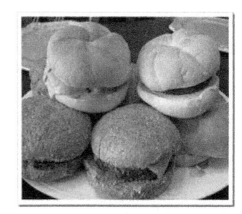

Preparations

Prepare ingredients and make salad in a large salad bowl. Store salad in the refrigerator until the hamburgers are ready to serve. Slice cheese for hamburgers.

Broil hamburger patty in the oven broiler or on a grill, until hamburger are cooked as desired. Season to taste with Bragg Organic Sprinkle and Bragg Liquid Aminos. Do not over cook. Place hamburgers on Ezekiel buns, place sliced tomatoes on hamburgers, followed by 2 to 4 leafs of Romaine lettuce to size of burger. Use a natural mustard or mayonnaise and serve.

Lemonade - Cut lemons into halves. Squeeze lemon juice into a 2 or 3-quart pitcher. Remove the seeds from the pitcher. Fill the pitcher with water. Sweeten the lemon water with Stevia to the desired level of sweetness

OPTIONAL; **Bragg** Healthy Vinaigrette. 2. Bragg Organic Hawaiian, Fat Free Dressing & Marinade. 3. Bragg Organic BraggBerry.

Ezekiel Bread and butter

http://bragg.com/products/bragg-organic-hawaiian-salad-dressing.html

SUMMARY

Is it a sin or a violation of God's principles to eat the kind of foods that promote a diseased condition? See Numbers 11:33 & 34. (Kibroth Hattaavah, Hebrew, meaning "Graves of Craving." Graves of Greed, Graves of lusting for meat.

God has established in 1 Corinthians 6:19 & 20 that your body is the temple of the Holy Ghost and it further states that ye are not your own. Verse 20 states that "For ye are bought with a price: therefore glorify God in your body, and in your Spirit, which is God's."

Clearly God is establishing in these two verses that our human bodies and Spirit belongs to God and is therefore the property of God's. Thus, it could be said that "you do not belong to yourself." As adults, God has blessed each of us as an agent, overseer, steward or trustee of the body each of us occupy. Accordingly as adults we have each been granted a divine responsibility to keep ourselves and our children well and free of food borne diseases.

Foods authorized by the Holy Scriptures refer to nine groups of foods consisting of sixty eight items for human consumption. Not including Ezekiel Bread from Ezekiel 4:9.

Man is made in God's image and likeness. Do you have any images of God suffering alzheimer's disease, cancer, diabetes, constipation or hemorrhoids? Its begs to question, is it a sin or a violation of God's principles to eat the kinds of foods that promote any diseased condition?

- Romans 11:21 refers to God spared not the natural branches... and
1 Corinthians 2:14 refers to natural man. In Foods authorized by the Holy Scriptures, God supplies natural foods for his natural human creation.

A significant number of health and wellness professionals agree, the further you drift from God's natural foods and the 90 essential nutrients needed to be disease free, you will be sailing onto a collision course into a food borne disease.

The recipes in this book are based on foods authorized by the Holy Bible.

Foods in the recipes not authorized by the Holy Bible are foods known to be nutritious and free of irritants. The ingredients in these recipes are designed to align natural foods from our natural God for consumption by God's natural men and women. The scope of these recipes and foods are somewhat limited and narrow based on the 69 foods named in the Holy Bible. Psalms 103:2 ... and forget not all his benefits:

- Matthew 7:13 – 14 Enter ye at the strait gate: for wide is the gate, and broad is the way, that leadeth to destruction, and many there be which go in thereat. Because strait is the gate, and narrow is the way, which leadeth unto life, and few there be that find it.

Creativity is encouraged using the 69 foods set forth in the Holy Bible within the preparation parameters' set forth by God. Cook and eat for life.

- Psalms 103:2 - 5 Bless the Lord, O my soul, and forget not all his benefits:
Who forgiveth all thine iniquities; who health all thy diseases;

Who redeemeth thy life from destruction; who crowneth thee with lovingkindness and tender mercies;
Who satisfieth thy mouth with good things; so that thy youth is renewed like the eagle's.

- **Revelation 22:10 - 13** And he saith unto me, seal not the sayings of the prophecy of this book: for the time is at hand.
He that is unjust, let him be unjust: and he which is filthy, let him be filthy still: and he that is righteous, let him be righteous still: and he that is holy, let him be holy still.
"And, behold, I come quickly; and my reward is with me, to give every man according as his work shall be."
I am Al'-pha and O-meg'-a the beginning and the end, the first and the last.

- **Proverbs 15:5** – A fool despiseth his father's instruction: but he that regardeth reproof is prudent.

Oh! What a mighty God we serve, and if we follow his directives, we will certainly be disease free.
Are you willing?

THE CENTERPOINT OF NUTRITION
90 Essential Nutrients

Youngevity products containing the 90 essential nutrients are listed below.

Beyond Tangy Tangerine Item # 23221 ....$48.50

Healthy Start Kit Item # 10245 ....$112.00

Classic 90 Pak Item # 10215 ....$79.00

Toddy 90 Pak Item # 10225 ....$77.75

Tropical 90 Pak Item # 10220 ....$70.00

Pig Pak Item # PigPak $150.00

Pig Pak Plus # PgPkPls $213.00

Bloomin Minerals, Soil Revitalizer – 40 LBS $67.00

Order at www.youngevityonline.com/oliversmithee or

Call Oliver Smith at 916-802-3482 to obtain preferred customer number. Preferred customer number required for wholesale pricing on products.

Recommended Reading

- The King James Version of the Holy Bible
- Where are the fathers?
- Black Gene Lies
- Dead Doctors Don't Lie
- God Bless America - Book
- Hell's Kitchen
- Immortality - Book
- Let's Play Herbal Doctors!
- Let's Play Doctors!
- Natural Cures, Saying Goodbye To Your Illness!
- Nature's First Law: The Raw Food Diet
- Passport to Aroma Therapy - Book
- Rare Earth, Forbidden Cures
- Wheat Grass, Nature's Finest Medicine
- Your Inner Body Adventure: A Trip of a Lifetime

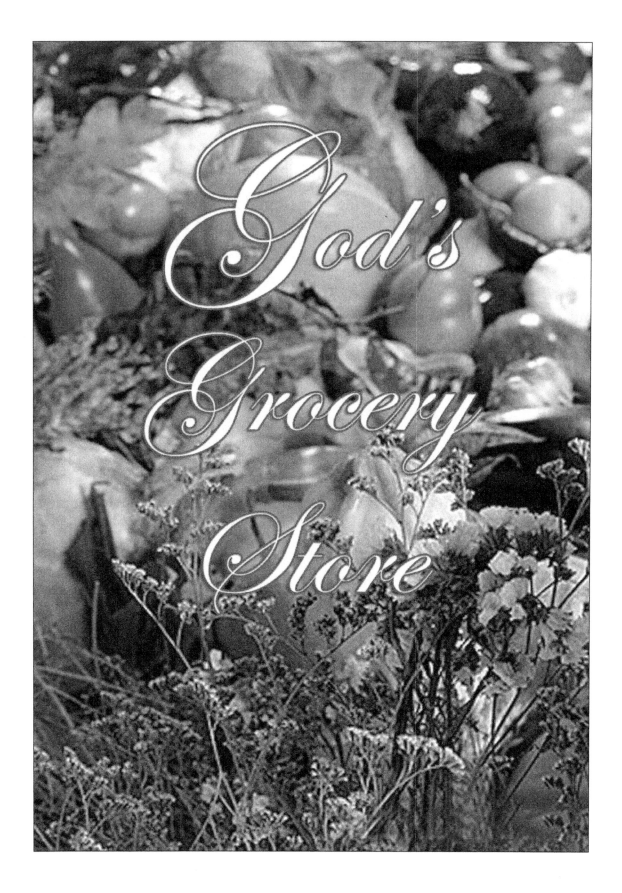

God's Grocery Store

Where women and men shop to acquire, obtain or purchase natural foods that are designed and created by God to keep us in the image and likeness of God as stated in; **Genesis 1:26 & 27.** God does not suffer food borne diseases and neither will we when we eat the natural foods that God put here for us to eat.

Where do we find God's natural foods?

- **1st choice** is to grow your own fruits, vegetables and meats. Now you are assured that your fruits, vegetables and meats are organic. And while you are at it, be sure to add Youngevity's Bloomin Minerals, Soil Revitalizer (Item # 64001) to the soil where the fruits and vegetables are to be grown.

- **2nd choice** is to seek and find farmers markets in your area. Always ask for organic or naturally grown fruits and vegetables. Always ask for meats that were fed a natural diet (grass fed). Ask for free range chickens and eggs, free range beef or lamb. Buy wild caught fish. Search for farmers markets online as well as local news papers and other local publications may be helpful.

- **3rd choice** is to take week-end and/or evening trips out to farm country seeking to find and create relationships with farmers who are producers and growers of organic and naturally grown fruits and vegetables. Online computer searches may be beneficial here as well.

- **4th choice** is to seek and find organic and/or natural grocery stores to supplement your food gathering processing from the first three choices.

God's Grocery Store by Pamela J. Johnson

God's Natural Spring Waters

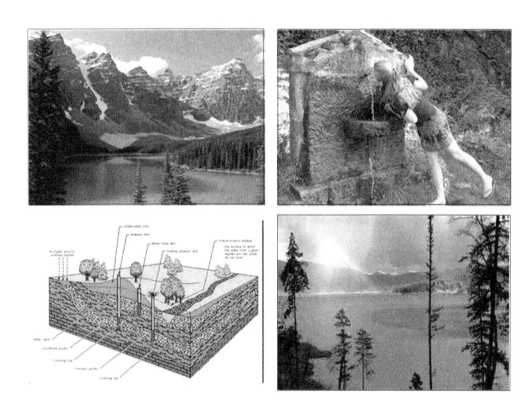

Isaiah 58:11 says, "And the Lord shall guide thee continually, and satisfy thy soul in drought, and make fat thy bones: and thou shall be like a watered garden, and like a spring of water, whose water fail not."

Revelation 21:6 says, "And he said unto me, it is done. I am Alpha and Omega, the beginning and the end. I will give unto him that is athirst of the fountain of the water of life freely."

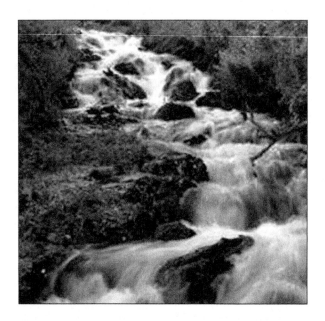
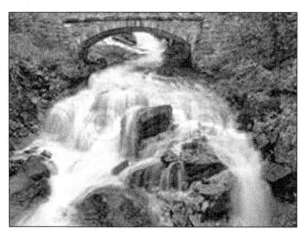
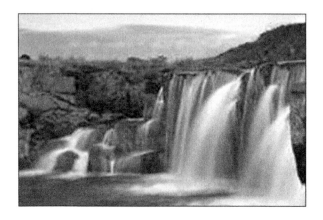

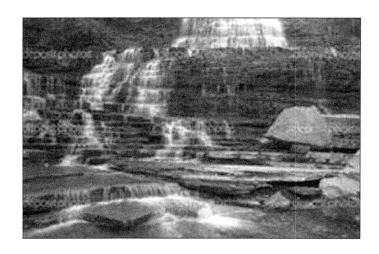

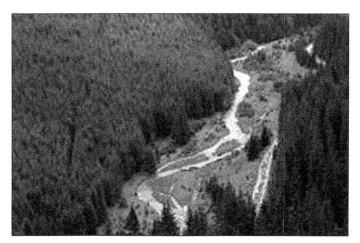

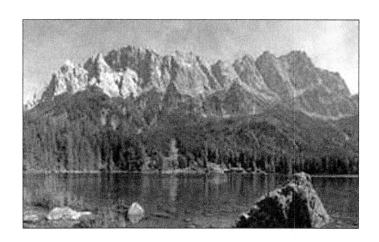

CLOSING PRAYER

Heavenly Father, we thank you for the Holy Bible and the covenants, laws, principles, and instructions set forth therein which guides us, your creations, towards a life that reflects the life you planned for us; when you made us in your image and likeness. We just pray Heavenly Father, that the readers of this book recognize that all of the Scriptures quoted regarding permitted and forbidden foods were taken from the King James version of the Holy Bible. We pray Father that you bless the readers of this book with the discipline to keep in their hearts, minds and Spirit 1st Corinthians 6:19-20, which clarifies that their bodies are the temples of the Holy Ghost and that their bodies and Spirits are God's. Father we pray that you glorify the readers of this book with the knowledge and understanding that they have a divine responsibility to keep the bodies that they are in stewardship of, free of food borne diseases, and that they not allow their taste buds to control their health.

Father, if it is your will, we ask for those who would take the time to read this book, that they connect the dots from this book to the Holy Bible and know that this book and the Holy Bible presents an opportunity for them to put their emotional, mental, physical, and spiritual well being back in the hands of their Lord and Savoir Jesus Christ. Father we just ask that the knowledge and understanding that the reader receives from this book and the Holy Bible will be passed on from this generation to multiple generations out into the future. Father, we pray that we glorify you Lord by making Genesis 6:3, a realization for all of your children. Heavenly Father, we pray these things in the name of Jesus. Amen!

And the Lord said, My spirit shall not always strive with man, for that he also is flesh: yet his days shall be an hundred and twenty years.
Genesis 6:3

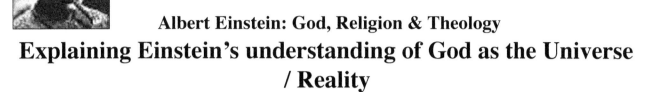

Albert Einstein: God, Religion & Theology
Explaining Einstein's understanding of God as the Universe / Reality

A knowledge of the existence of something we cannot penetrate, of the manifestations of the profoundest reason and the most radiant beauty - it is this knowledge and this emotion that constitute the truly religious attitude; in this sense, and in this alone, I am a deeply religious man. (**Albert Einstein**)

I do not believe in a personal God and I have never denied this but have expressed it clearly. If something is in me which can be called religious then it is the unbounded admiration for the structure of the world so far as our science can reveal it. (**Albert Einstein, 1954**)

I believe in Spinoza's God who reveals himself in the orderly harmony of what exists, not in a God who concerns himself with the fates and actions of human beings. (**Albert Einstein**)

Ecclesiastes 12:13 says, "Let us hear the conclusion of the whole matter: Fear God, and keep his commandments: for this is the whole *duty* of man."

God blessed man & woman with air to breath, water to drink, sun light to promote human growth, why would he NOT bless man & woman with food that would keep man & woman free of food borne disease!!!!!

Oliver Smith

"And God blessed them, and God said unto them, Be fruitful, and multiply, and replenish the earth, and subdue it: and have dominion over the fish of the sea, and over the fowl of the air, and over every living thing that moveth upon the earth."

Genesis 1:28

"And God said, Behold, I have given you every herb bearing seed, which is upon the face of all the earth, and every tree, in the which is the fruit of a tree yielding seed; to you it shall be for meat."

Genesis 1:29

"A fool despiseth his father's instruction: but he that regardeth reproof is prudent"

Proverbs 15:5

"Give instruction to a wise man, and he will be yet wiser: teach a just man, and he will increase in learning."

Proverbs 9:9

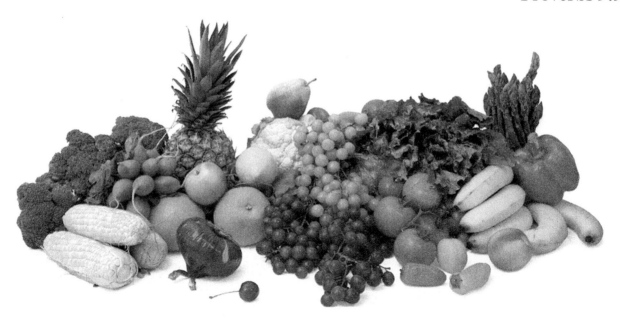

CPSIA information can be obtained
at www.ICGtesting.com
Printed in the USA
LVOW02s1344120616

492278LV00035B/1101/P